ROYAL COLLEGE
OF PHYSICIANS AND SURGEONS OF CANADA | CanMEDS

CanMEDS Physician Health Guide

A Practical Handbook for Physician Health and Well-being

Editors:

Derek Puddester, MD MEd FRCPC
Associate Professor, Department of Psychiatry
Director, Faculty Wellness Program, Faculty of Medicine
University of Ottawa

Leslie Flynn, MD MMus CCFP FRCPC
Associate Dean, Postgraduate Medical Education
Associate Professor, Departments of Psychiatry and Family Medicine
Queen's University

Jordan Cohen, MD FRCPC
Assistant Clinical Professor, Department of Psychiatry, Faculty of Medicine
Director of Student Affairs, Undergraduate Medical Education
University of Calgary

Series Editor
Jason R. Frank, MD MA(Ed) FRCPC
Associate Director, Office of Education
Royal College of Physicians and Surgeons of Canada

CanMEDS Physician Health Guide

A Practical Handbook for Physician Health and Well-being

The Royal College of Physicians and Surgeons of Canada
774 Echo Drive
Ottawa, Ontario K1S 5N8 Canada
Telephone: 613-730-8177
Toll-Free: 1-800-668-3740
Fax: 613-730-3707
Website: royalcollege.ca/canmeds
E-mail: canmeds@rcpsc.edu

Printed in Ottawa, Ontario, Canada. First Printing

Cover photos
Main image: iStockphoto LP
Additional images by Angela Hubbard at the Ottawa Hospital.
Photos throughout by Angela Hubbard and iStockphoto LP.

ISBN: 978-1-926588-03-2

How to reference this document:

Puddester D, Flynn L, Cohen J. 2009. CanMEDS physician health guide: A practical handbook for physician health and well-being. Ottawa: The Royal College of Physicians and Surgeons of Canada.

Dedicated to Michael F. Myers, MD FRCPC
Canada's physician health pioneer

Foreword: Time for a practical handbook for physician health and well-being

Jason R. Frank, MD MA(Ed) FRCPC; Jon Cormier, MA; Cynthia Abbott, MPl; and Sarah Taber, MHA/MGSS

"Physician health" is an emerging field in medicine, and this book marks another milestone in its development. As described by Puddester in the Introduction, physician health used to be a euphemism for a clinician with a substance abuse problem. We have come a long, long way from those days. Today, the field has expanded in scope and depth. We live in an era in which there is a world shortage of health professionals, and no prospect for relief in our practice lifetime. More than ever, we need every available health professional to possess the healthy lives that they work to promote in their patients. In an era of increasing intensity, accountability, upheaval, and scarcity in health care, we need to support sustainable practices for those in the health professions too. Numerous pioneering leaders have developed physician health, not only as an area of practice, but also a field of scholarship, and moreover, an imperative. In this book, Puddester, Flynn, and Cohen et al, answer this call. Leading practitioners and scholars have assembled their insights into a publication with a unique niche: an accessible, useful, ready resource for those thinking or teaching about physician health and well-being. From addictions to zeitgebers, from career planning to financial planning, *The CanMEDS Physician Health Guide* is a handy source for information.

The CanMEDS Physician Health Guide is the latest resource from the Royal College of Physicians and Surgeons of Canada's national faculty development program. This program supports the teaching and assessment of the CanMEDS Roles in medicine by creating resources and Train-the-trainer Workshops to support each of the seven identified domains of physician competence. *The CanMEDS Physician Health Guide* relates specifically to the Professional Role, a domain that includes the ability of physicians to demonstrate a commitment to physician health and sustainable practice.

As Professionals, physicians are committed to the health and well-being of individuals and society through ethical practice, profession-led regulation, and high personal standards of behaviour. However, by dedicating so much of themselves to the health and caring of others, physicians can lose sight of their own health needs. *The CanMEDS Physician Health Guide* was created with the idea that having healthy physicians is a necessary ingredient for excellence in health care.

The CanMEDS Physician Health Guide is an introduction to the broad scope of issues that make up physician health. As a toolkit, this publication is an easy-to-access resource which all physicians can use to pursue better physician health. Using real-world situations and scenarios, this guide will help physicians discover practical and useful strategies for introducing and promoting physical, emotional, and spiritual well-being.

The topics covered throughout *The CanMEDS Physician Health Guide* were identified by a panel of experts—physicians who work with other physicians who have health concerns. Content experts were challenged to present their topic in a simple two-page spread that introduces readers to the topic, provides a sample case, and additional references for further reading. As a result, readers can quickly access information on any topic area and find a succinct summary of information along with the tools for further exploration.

What is the purpose of *The CanMEDS Physician Health Guide*?

As the nature of contemporary health care evolves and develops, so does the role of physician. The term "physician health" has become one of the cornerstone ideas to improving the delivery of health care, with the thesis that healthy medical practitioners are a necessary ingredient in offering a higher quality of care. Medicine can be a very rewarding career but it is also a very demanding profession. As this guide shows the hazards to physician health are wide ranging – from poor nutrition to problems with finances to stress management – these are the issues that can and do affect all physicians at some stage in their careers.

Throughout the handbook, each chapter acts as an introduction to a subject and provides practical information for understanding the issue. The chapters are created to be accessible within the busy schedule many physicians maintain. This handbook not only creates awareness to the wide-ranging factors involved in maintaining a sustainable practice but presents easy-to-follow solutions to many of the issues surrounding physician health.

Who created the handbook?

The CanMEDS Physician Health Guide has been created by practicing physicians from across Canada and international locations who are subject matter experts in the areas each has written on.

How is the information presented?

At its core this is a practical guide for dealing with the issues that make up physician health. *The CanMEDS Physician Health Guide* is thematically organized into 11 Sections that cover the main areas of physician health, including a section that presents many of the practical resources currently available to assist physicians and their own health needs. Each section is divided into chapters which present the specific elements that make up the larger themes. The chapters are presented in a two-page layout complete with specific learning objectives, a practical case and case resolution, the core information on the subject, key resources and reflective exercises.

CanMEDS Professional Role

Definition

As Professionals, physicians are committed to the health and well-being of individuals and society through ethical practice, profession-led regulation, and high personal standards of behaviour.

Key Competencies

Physicians are able to…

1. Demonstrate a commitment to their patients, profession, and society through ethical practice;
2. Demonstrate a commitment to their patients, profession, and society through participation in profession-led regulation;
3. Demonstrate a commitment to physician health and sustainable practice.

The goal of this publication is to have a resource that not only describes what makes up physician health, but to have an easy to access handbook for dealing with physician health issues directly. There is a quick reference index at the end of the book made up of key terms and issues for dealing with physician health needs and each section is colour coded, so finding specific information is quick and simple.

Who is this handbook for?

The Royal College is committed to creating resources for medical education, physician competence and quality care. *The CanMEDS Physician Health Guide* has been designed for multiple stakeholders, including:

Medical educators

Medical educators will find a resource on the principles of physician health. *The CanMEDS Physician Health Guide* introduces the myriad of topics that make up physician health, well-being, and sustainability. When creating curriculum or trying to answer questions that come up during a teaching session, *The CanMEDS Physician Health Guide* is there to introduce a subject, provide key information on the topic, present a case and case resolution, and to provide key resources and further reading on the topic. This guide expands upon the Professional Role from the CanMEDS Framework and can be used to highlight the complexities of physician health and sustainable practice.

Teachers

The CanMEDS Physician Health Guide is also a resource for front-line clinical teachers. The easy to access format is intended to facilitate bedside teaching. The cases are derived from evidence of patients' needs, from practicing physicians' perspectives, from content experts and from empirical research. This guide helps teachers ask effective educational questions that explore the variety of aspects that make up physician health and lead to sustainable practice.

Trainees and students

The CanMEDS Physician Health Guide is aimed to directly address the learning needs of medical students and residents. Although the guide provides information for physicians throughout their careers the information is presented to show students and residents many of the everyday issues that can (and do) affect physician health. Along with presenting learning moments, this publication provides practical advice for those in training to help manage their own health in the form of available resources, practical advice, and key references for each topic.

Practicing physicians

The CanMEDS Physician Health Guide is a simple resource for physicians treating other physicians. This guide presents the "bigger picture" for all the phases of a physician's lifecycle and the issues surrounding physician health. The basis for all CanMEDS products is that they are created by physicians for physicians. The information and cases are based on scenarios that practicing physicians will recognize. Similarly the resources identified throughout the handbook make this guide a powerful tool for maintaining one's own health.

The authors and editors have done an outstanding job in bringing this together. We trust you find it useful.

Key reference

Frank JR, ed. 2005. Professional. In *The CanMEDS 2005 Physician Competency Framework*. Ottawa: The Royal College, 23–4. Last retrieved August 19, 2009: rcpsc.medical.org/canmeds/CanMEDS2005/CanMEDS2005_e.pdf.

Table of contents

Table of Contents

Table of Contents

Editorial Team

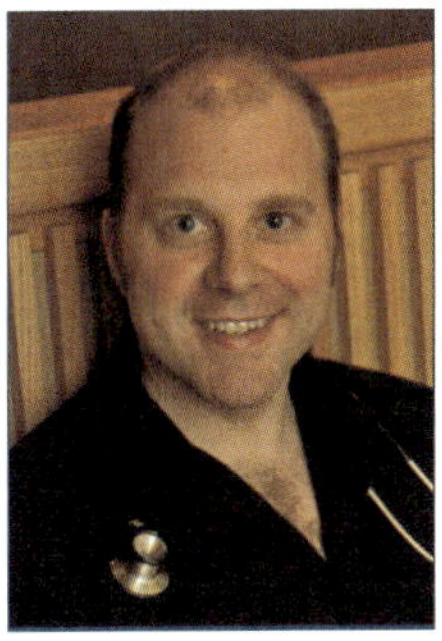

Derek Puddester, MD MEd FRCPC

Dr. Puddester completed his undergraduate training in English/Russian Studies and Medicine at Memorial University of Newfoundland. He completed a Psychiatry Residency at McMaster University and a Fellowship in Child Psychiatry at uOttawa. He is the Medical Leader of the Behavioural Neurosciences and Consultation-Liaison Team at the Children's Hospital of Eastern Ontario. Dr. Puddester is also the Director of Continuing Medical Education and Professional Development for the Department of Psychiatry at CHEO. Dr. Puddester is an Associate Professor at uOttawa's Faculty of Medicine where he also serves as the Director of the Faculty Wellness Program. Dr. Puddester's educational and research work focuses on physician health, healthy work environments, e-learning, and curriculum theory and development. The Canadian Association of Interns and Residents has recognized his leadership in physician health by creating the *Dr. Derek Puddester Resident Well-Being Award* which is given annually to a person or program that has made a significant contribution to the improvement of resident health and wellness. He is a proud Newfoundlander, parent, partner and son. Ask him about geocaching, the value of play, and power of actualized ideas.

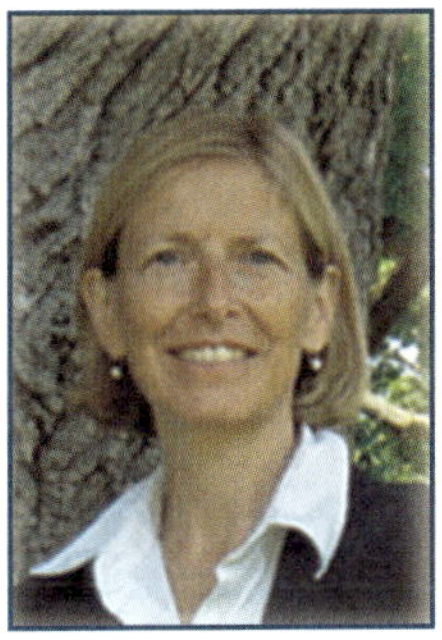

Leslie Flynn, MD MMus CCFP FRCPC

After receiving her undergraduate degree in Music from Queen's University and a Master's in Music from the University of Toronto in 1982, Dr. Flynn returned to Queen's where she receive her MD in 1987 and undertook her postgraduate medical education training. She became certified as a Family Physician in 1988 and subsequently as a psychiatrist in 1995. She then began her professional career at Queen's University when she was cross-appointed to the Departments of Family Medicine and Psychiatry in the role of Family Medicine Liaison Psychiatrist. She has held roles as Director of the Continuing Medical Education program, Postgraduate Program Director and the Director of Psychotherapy in the Department of Psychiatry. Dr. Flynn is currently an Associate Professor in the Departments of Psychiatry and Family Medicine and the Associate Dean of Postgraduate Medical Education at Queen's University.

Dr. Flynn has received departmental awards for *Excellent Leadership in Education and Dedication to the Ideals of the Department* as well as the *Annual Staff Excellence in Teaching Award.* She has conducted research in physician health, the Role of Health Advocate, interprofessional education and the scholarship of teaching and learning.

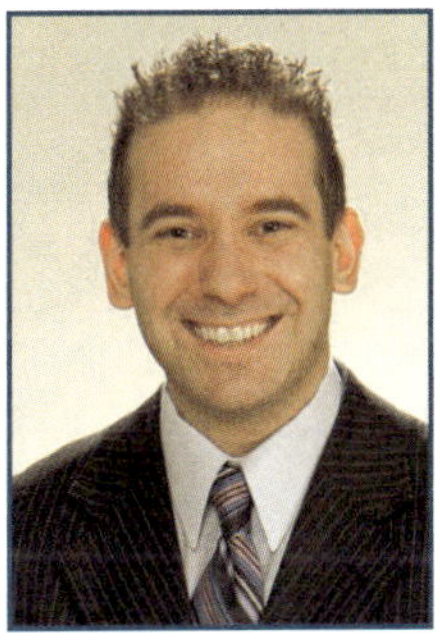

Jordan Cohen, MD FRCPC

Dr. Cohen is currently an Assistant Clinical Professor in the Department of Psychiatry of the Faculty of Medicine at the University of Calgary, where he completed both his residency and undergraduate medical training. He is also the Director of Student Affairs of Undergraduate Medical Education and Chair of *The Physicianship Course* for the Faculty of Medicine at the University of Calgary. His educational and research work focuses on balancing medicine, physician health and professionalism.

Dr. Cohen is a child and adolescent psychiatrist appointed as Medical Director of NW Family and Adolescent/Child Services, Consultant Psychiatrist at the Young Adult Program (Foothills Hospital), and Consulting Psychiatrist at the Arnika Centre for individuals with developmental disabilities. He is also a board member of the Physician Health Monitoring Program for the Alberta College of Physicians and Surgeons.

Dr. Cohen has received multiple awards including: the *Canadian Medical Association's CMA Award for Young Leaders* (Early Career Physician) 2009; the Canadian Association of Interns and Residents, *Dr. Derek Puddester Resident Well Being Award* 2006 for his contributions to resident health; the *Department of Psychiatry's Postgraduate Clinical Education Award* 2008 in recognition of outstanding contribution in the area of postgraduate clinical education; and the *Department of Psychiatry's Postgraduate Research Award for Part-time Faculty* 2008 in recognition of outstanding research contributions in Psychiatry.

A. Goals and objectives of this guide

The vast majority of today's physicians entered their profession after considerable reflection, years of academic preparation, and in the face of significant competition and challenge. The intellectual, emotional, physical and social demands of medical training are rigorous, as are the professional and personal demands of practice. The good news is that most physicians thrive in their work environments, are strong and healthy, practise excellent strategies to safeguard their own well-being, and enjoy long and healthy lives. When physicians' personal well-being and professional commitment are in balance, positive synergies result that sustain them in their healing role, to the benefit of patients and the health care system as a whole.

And yet the phrase physician health seems not to convey that common reality. For many decades it was a euphemistic reference to struggles with addiction. Slowly, provincial medical associations and colleges began to develop innovative programs that provided treatment and support services primarily for issues related to substance abuse. However, physician health programs have evolved dramatically in recent years in response to demand for a range of services to address issues ranging from depression, anxiety and suicidal ideation to disruptive behaviour, risk of relapse and family discord. The growth of these programs has been consistent across Canada, and physician organizations continue to support a deeper understanding of "physician health."

In collaboration with other stakeholders and partners across the country, the Royal College of Physicians and Surgeons of Canada is now taking a leadership role in the field of physician health. The CanMEDS project has modernized Canadian specialty medicine and is being adopted in many countries in response to the increasing complexity of contemporary health care delivery. Although, as is the case with many physician competencies, aspects of physician health can readily fit into many CanMEDS roles, the College has anchored it within the Professional Role. Specifically, as professionals, physicians are committed to the health and well-being of individuals and society through ethical practice, profession-led regulation, and high personal standards of behaviour." The key competencies of this role demand that physicians:

- *Demonstrate a commitment to their patients, profession and society through ethical practice;*
- *Demonstrate a commitment to their patients, profession, and society through participation in profession-led regulation; and*
- *Demonstrate a commitment to physician health and sustainable practice.*

This handbook is designed to help educators and learners better understand the broad meaning of "physician health," to discover practical strategies to promote professional health and to apply such knowledge to real-world situations. It is not meant to be an academic exercise, but rather to form part of a practical toolkit of resources that Canadian physicians can access and apply as they see fit. Readers can use this handbook to explore their own questions and needs, educators can draw upon it as a resource for teaching and learning programs, and investigators may find it helpful in identifying avenues for research in physician health.

Topic areas were identified by a panel of experts who work in the trenches with physicians presenting with health concerns. Content experts were invited to cover these topics—including sample cases, strategies and solutions, references, and reflective exercises—in a succinct format that would allow readers to access information quickly while encouraging further exploration.

It has been an honour to work on this project on behalf of the Royal College, and I am grateful to my coeditors, the brilliant and enthusiastic volunteer contributors, the project team, and the many colleagues and learners who provided feedback and guidance along the way. Our profession truly is wonderful, and it shines the brightest when we collaborate to create powerful and meaningful change.

Derek Puddester, MD MEd FRCPC
Associate Professor, Psychiatry
Director, Faculty Wellness Program
University of Ottawa
Correspondence: drpuddester@me.com

Key reference

Frank JR, ed. 2005. Professional. In *The CanMEDS 2005 Physician Competency Framework*. Ottawa: The Royal College, 23–4.

B. A conceptual framework for physician health

Derek Puddester, MD MEd FRCPC

Objectives

This section will

- articulate the basic concepts of physician health and sustainability,
- introduce a potential conceptual framework for physician health, and
- describe critical aspects of such a framework in detail for the reader.

Case

A resident entered medicine after volunteering at an Easter Seals camp for many summers and discovering a love of working with children with disabilities. With divorced parents, and not having a strong relationship with either of them; this early experience taught the resident to be independent, contributed to some social isolation and triggered a certain ineptness in interpersonal relationships. By choosing a specialty the resident found the work stimulating, the hours reasonable, and the job opportunities broad. Until recently, life has been highly focused on training, but now the resident has begun to realize that they are lonely. This resident has few friends, has not dated anyone in several years, and has no real interests outside of training. The resident wonders if they are depressed, even though their mental and physical health have previously been excellent.

Introduction

Conceptual frameworks can help us to quickly grasp the relationships among complex ideas and to clarify the terms of a discussion. This guidebook uses such a framework to propose a common understanding of the essential components of physician health, and in fact to broaden the definition of physician health. This framework is represented schematically in the figure below. The ensuing discussion will describe its main components.

Systemic issues

Physicians are educated and work within a medical system that has an identity, a regulatory code, a set of expectations, unique strengths and many challenges. It is important to acknowledge that physicians have little immediate control over "the system," and to a considerable degree are controlled by it. However, that system has strengths that contribute to physicians' professional health. Canadian health care embodies generally held values of universal access to health services, protection of society's most vulnerable members, and the notion of collective contributions to the health of the nation. Physicians are thus part of the very fabric that defines the Canadian ethos, and this fact in itself sustains many of us during our most challenging hours.

At the same time, the Canadian health care system presents many challenges. Well over a million Canadians have no physician, and thousands of physicians are working more hours per week than is permitted for long-distance truck drivers, air traffic controllers or airline pilots. The demand for health care simply outstrips resources, and most physicians respond by working harder, longer and in more complex environments.

FIGURE 1.
Conceptual Framework for Physician Health

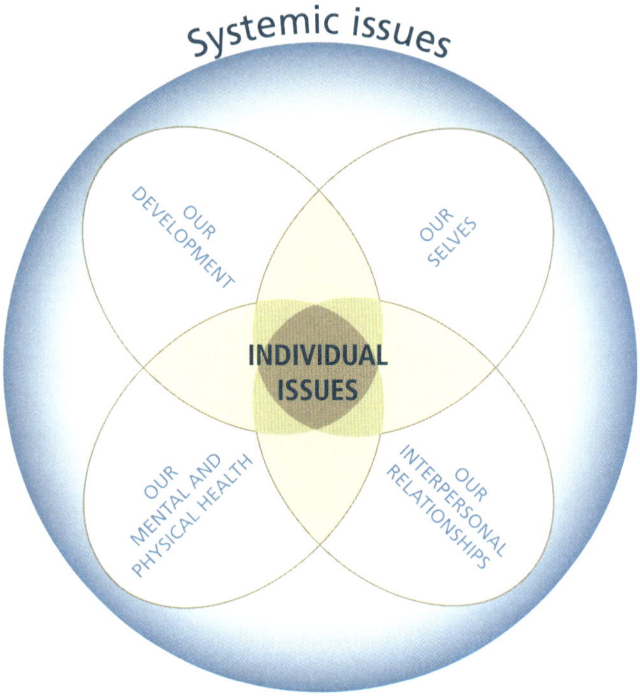

Physician enfranchisement is another complex area, given the position of physicians as private practitioners or contractors. Our advocacy skills are often put to the test in our relationships with governments, hospitals, universities or other large and powerful institutions. Yet the resulting exchange, negotiation, debate and interchange helps build a better system for all. It is essential that such communication not only continue, but be encouraged. Disenfranchised physicians tend to use their advocacy skills for only so long before they feel forced into a difficult choice such as leaving their practice or, worse, simply burning out. The system and the profession need to acknowledge that they nurture and sustain each other, and that they achieve far more synergistically than they do as adversaries. Physicians can promote their own health and well-being by being actively involved in medical policy and decision-making, volunteering with their medical associations and colleges, and using their advocacy skills to promote a vision of a healthy Canada for all.

Individual issues

Preserving the self. We are all more than what others see, or think they see. The physician's white coat serves many purposes, including facilitating professional detachment from the tragedy, horror and pain encountered on a daily basis. Yet it is important that we remain in touch with who we are, how we feel, our methods of responding and reacting to our world, and our ideas about what makes us healthy—or not. The interplay of the personal and professional self is constant, sometimes complicated, and useful. Our own stories colour and, ideally, can make our responses more compassionate to similar stories encountered in our patients. The better we understand our inner selves, the better we can manage our own strengths and vulnerabilities as our professional selves develop and mature.

Mental and physical health. Mental health is a complex issue for many Canadians. People with mental illness still experience social stigma, and even within the house of medicine mental illness engenders misunderstanding and fear. Although attitudes are changing, the medical profession must continue to address the stigmatization of mental illness as an essential aspect of promoting mental health for all.

Rates of common mental illnesses such as anxiety and depression are higher among physicians than among the general Canadian population. At certain times—such as during training, major professional or personal transitions, or when dealing with complaints or litigation—physicians are particularly vulnerable to mental illness. By openly talking about such vulnerabilities, ensuring safe and rapid access to support services and programs, and promoting resilience, medical schools and physician health programs can help individuals safeguard their own wellness and remain in practice or training.

The maintenance of good physical health is no less important. For example, weight gain is common issue among students and residents and usually occurs in the context of a shift in priorities that causes exercise routines and good eating habits to lapse. The challenges posed by chronic health conditions are also important to acknowledge, as are the needs of trainees with disabilities. Students and residents with disabilities have rights that require respect and consideration, and training systems need to make reasonable accommodation to ensure that they have equitable opportunities to achieve certification and enter practice.

Interpersonal relationships. Medicine is a profession based on interpersonal relationships. The ability to form a meaningful connection with patients and families is paramount, as is the ability to forge productive collegial relationships with other physicians, allied health professionals and health system stakeholders. Although "people skills" such as honesty, genuineness, humour, empathy, insight and compassion are typical of most physicians, other traits, such as perfectionism and defensiveness, can get in the way of interpersonal relationships to the detriment of patient care. Beyond the workplace, some physicians struggle to remain connected to friends and family and to sustain personal pursuits while juggling the demands of their career. However, it is important to maintain non-professional ties. Multiple social connections promote emotional resilience and good health, while isolation fosters burnout and depression.

Lifelong development. Like all other human beings, physicians are in a continuous process of personal change. Their physical selves need care and maintenance, their sexual self matures and evolves, and their use of health services increases. In general, mental resilience increases over time while vulnerabilities retreat. Personal relationships grow deeper and more meaningful at the same time as they change. In short, physicians are always growing and developing. Stagnation is rare, and where it exists may signal ill-health. For physicians as for others, many of life's challenges centre on transitions: from residency to practice, from one career stage to another, from one personal milestone to the next. And, for physicians as for everyone, an important component of coping with transitions is to maintain a sense of optimism and to make lifestyle choices that are conducive to healthy self-care.

Case resolution

In the absence of other symptoms, it is unlikely that the resident is mentally ill. However, it seems that early life experiences led to a pessimistic view of adult relationships and for the resident to be overly self-reliant. By sacrificing many aspects of normal development (e.g., friendships, dating, intimacy) to ensure independent survival, and compensating for the lack of a "personal life" this resident developed a strong work ethic and became consumed by professional commitments. Professionally, this has led to isolation from colleagues and perhaps patients; personally, it has resulted in loneliness and potential despair.

In some ways, the resident needs to complete adolescence and early adulthood. The resident should reflect on their self, identify two or three activities to pursue during free time (e.g., sports, recreation, volunteering) and try to cultivate friendships and relationships slowly but meaningfully. By working toward building personal connections with others, the resident will learn more about their own temperament and be more aware of their authentic self. In turn, this connection and insight will help promote self-resilience and promote a sustainable practice.

Key reference

University of Ottawa, the University of Ontario Institute of Technology and Durham College. *Conceptual Framework Learning Object.* Last retrieved July 17, 2009: innovation.dc-uoit.ca/cloe/lo/cf/CF_LO_content.html.

C. The Professional Role and physician health

Leslie Flynn, MD MMus CCFP FRCPC

Objectives

This section will

- consider the meaning of medical professionalism,
- describe how aspects of the Professional Role can give rise to stress, and
- propose ways to build resiliency in the Professional Role.

Case

While working in a hospital, a fourth-year resident is contacted by a community pharmacist who wants to clarify the dose of narcotic prescribed for a physician colleague and friend. The resident is taken aback, as they have never written such a prescription for this person. The pharmacist confirms that the resident's name and signature are on the prescription and that this is the same person who provided prescriptions for the physician in the past when filled at this pharmacy.

Introduction

The process of becoming a physician is arduous and involves more than acquiring a career and a livelihood. It brings those who follow this path great personal benefit, including the privilege of entering a prestigious and honourable profession. The inception of medicine as a profession dates to the Hippocratic Oath, which was established in the fourth century B.C. as a moral code for all who wished to practise the physician's art. Since then, society has relied on medical practitioners to be trustworthy and to care for their patients according to an accepted high standard. They bring expertise, critical thinking, sound judgment and compassion to their work. They make a commitment to address disinterestedly the problems of individual patients, communities and society as a whole, according to the accepted principles and practices of their discipline.

What does it mean to be a professional?

Professionalism is difficult to define concisely and thoroughly. Many concepts are implied by the term, some of which are more familiar than others. Medical professionals are expected to have mastered a complex body of knowledge and skills, to adhere to a code of ethics, to communicate well, and to practise medicine as a humanistic "art" as well as a "science." As professionals, physicians are expected to:

- demonstrate and uphold the values of clinical competence,
- embrace appropriate attitudes and behaviours,
- act with integrity,
- be altruistic, and
- promote the public good.

These commitments form the basis of a social contract by which physicians are accountable to society; in return, the profession enjoys the privilege of self-regulation.

The figure below represents one definition of professionalism. It identifies the elements that are typically considered essential to the physician's Professional Role.

Figure 2. Defining professionalism

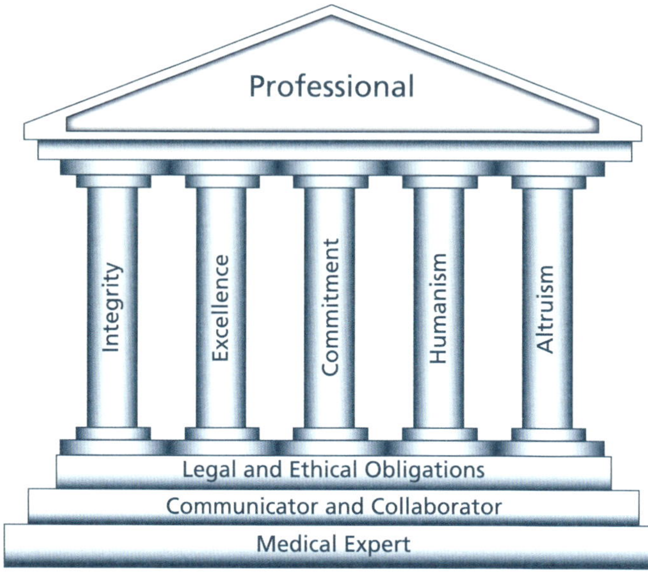

Responsibilities and stress

The principles of professionalism are relevant to the entire career path of physicians, applying to their behaviour as medical students, residents and practitioners. With membership in the medical profession comes tremendous responsibility. Society's expectations of physicians are great, and the challenge of meeting them is compounded by the rapid pace of change and the increasing complexity of today's health care environment. Most physicians experience stressful working environments, and learning to cope with stress has always been a normal part of medical training and practice. Although we know that a certain degree of stress can enhance an individual's performance, stress of a certain nature, magnitude or duration can lead to psychological distress, impaired health and suboptimal performance.

A community of physicians

Neighbourhood Watch is an well-known organization established to help keep communities safe. Community members join the organization and pledge to watch out for one another. They attempt to protect one another from harm. Would it be possible to establish a similar model in medicine? Could we establish a Community of Physicians who take responsibility for protecting one another in a simple and neighbourly way? Creating caring communities has the potential to bring physicians together and to make an important contribution to improving their lives.

This recognition, along with an awareness of the importance of physician sustainability in maintaining a healthy medical workforce, has led to the inclusion of physicians' maintenance of their own health and well-being as a necessary component of their professional role. In Canada, the recognition that physician well-being is essential to the effective practise of medicine is reflected in the *Code of Ethics* of the Canadian Medical Association (CMA) and in the Royal College of Physicians and Surgeons of Canada's CanMEDS Professional competency description.

The CMA *Code of Ethics* stipulates that a physician must practise the art and science of medicine competently, with integrity and without impairment, and that it is incumbent upon physicians to promote and maintain their own health and well-being.

The Royal College CanMEDS Framework identifies that a competent physician demonstrates a commitment to physician health and sustainable practice. This entails: (a) balancing personal and professional priorities to ensure personal health and a sustainable practice; (b) striving to heighten personal and professional awareness and insight; (c) recognizing other professionals in need and responding appropriately.

Reflection

What physicians have been your models of medical professionalism? What is it about them that captures the spirit of the profession? How do they behave? How do they interact with colleagues, patients and families? Think about how you use these models as your guide.

Professionalism and physician health

Although aspects of self-care are now considered an integral component of medical professionalism, they are often neglected by physicians. In part, this results from the very attributes that are valued in physicians. For example, altruism has the potential to lead to self-neglect, given that physicians are expected to put their patients' interests before their own. Physicians are also expected to be autonomous, and may not be encouraged to acknowledge their own health vulnerabilities or to seek help when they need it. We know that physicians, as a group, do not avail themselves of a regular source of health care. Indeed, physicians may resort to self-prescribing. When feeling stressed and overwhelmed, physicians may turn to the use of substances as a means of coping. Physicians feel unable to access help—either for the originating problem, or for the resulting dependency—without feeling ashamed and humiliated.

This tendency to deny vulnerability is pervasive among physicians. Hence, when physicians see one of their colleagues struggle with a personal or professional problem, the inclination is to say nothing. This neglect of tending to the needs of colleagues heightens the silence around physician illness and impairment. Additionally, regulatory authorities and their health history requisitions inadvertently add to the desire to keep one's problems private. The fear of exposure and the potential for consequences regarding licensure lead physicians to deny their need for assistance. These conflicts pose significant challenges to meeting the physician's professional responsibility.

Summary

Being a member of the profession of medicine is a desirable and highly rewarding accomplishment. The professional requirements of a physician are tremendously demanding. It is a physician's duty to behave according to the high standards of the profession. This includes being diligent in attending to one's own health and well-being while also watching over one's brothers and sisters in the community of medicine.

Case resolution

The resident is shocked and states they are not their colleague's physician nor did they write the prescription. They are not sure what to do next and they call their provincial health program for advice that is helpful and supportive.

Key references

Canadian Medical Association. 2004. *Code of Ethics.*[policy]. Ottawa: The CMA.

Frank JR, ed. 2005. *The CanMEDS 2005 Physician Competency Framework. Better Standards. Better Physicians. Better Care.* Ottawa: The Royal College of Physicians and Surgeons of Canada.

D. Physician health: A business case

Edgardo Pérez, MD MPH FRCPC and Karen J. Parsons

Objectives

This section will

- examine the importance of physician health to the quality and efficiency of health care delivery, and
- discuss the impact that gender and generational differences have on a business model for physician health.

> **Case**
>
> A third-year resident has been calling in sick for several days over the last two rotations. This has come to the attention of the program director through preceptors, who have both been practising medicine for over 25 years.

Introduction

A survey conducted by the Canadian Medical Association (CMA) in 2003 yielded the following rather alarming findings:

- 46 per cent of Canadian physicians are in an advanced stage of burnout, (CMA 2007)
- 77 per cent feel that they do not have enough time to get everything done (Lamaire and Wallace 2008), and
- only 47 per cent report that they have a balanced life. (Lamaire and Wallace 2008)

Further research commissioned by the CMA and the Institute of Neurosciences, Mental Health and Addiction, showed the link between work organization and mental health problems among physicians (Quality Worklife 2007). As former CMA president Dr. Brian Day has stated, "The health of Canada's doctors is crucial to the provision of high-quality health care for our patients and it is why the CMA has made 'Physician Health' one of the organization's five key priority areas." (CMA 2007)

Among the respondents to the National Physician Survey for 2007, (CFPC et al 2007)

- 13 per cent had been absent from work in the previous year as a result of illness or disability,
- 2 per cent had been ill from work-related stress, and
- 4 per cent had been absent because of maternity or paternity leave (a quarter of these absences were 4 weeks or less).

In 2003–04, 34 per cent of the almost 2000 resident physicians who participated in the Happy Doc pilot survey reported that their daily lives were "quite a bit" to "extremely" stressful. Coping mechanisms included alcohol and drug use. 24 per cent of respondents said they would pursue another career if they could, and 53 per cent said that they had experienced intimidation and harassment more than once during their training. In addition,

- 18 per cent rated their mental health as fair or poor,
- 23 per cent reported that they had experienced an emotional or mental health problem during residency, and
- 36 per cent reported that they did not have a family physician (Cohen 2004).

Stress factors that affect physician well-being include

- fear that seeking help would have a negative effect on one's career,
- expecting to be able to "do it all" and patients "expecting it all,"
- excessive workload and too little control of work situation,
- worries about potential medico-legal liability, and
- being on call and working shifts (CMA 2003).

On this last point, the CMA cites survey findings that 76 per cent of doctors do on-call work, 36 per cent say that their total monthly on-call hours are stressful or highly stressful and 29 per cent say that their on-call responsibilities are too onerous (CMA 2003).

Physicians are subject to a variety of workplace hazards, including exposure to infectious diseases and, occasionally, abuse and harassment by patients. These threats can contribute to job stress. The risks for disease and injury are as high—or higher—for physicians as for other workers.

The economic benefits of promoting physician health should not be overlooked. For example, the finding by Buchbinder and colleagues in 1999 that recruitment and replacement costs for individual primary care physicians were $236,393 for general/family practice and $245,128 for general internal medicine, highlights the fiscal impact of physician turnover (Gautam 2008).

Physicians are key to reversing current trends in the development and onset of major depressive disorders among men and women in their prime working years, (Wilkerson 2008) which according to the Centre for Addiction and Mental Health now cost Canada more than $51 billion a year in lost productive capacity.

Patient safety

Of obvious concern in relation to physician health and wellness is the ability of practitioners to treat their patients in a timely, consistent and safe manner. Physicians who are struggling with unmanaged mental or physical problems put both themselves and their patients at risk.

Many of the participants in a study conducted in Calgary reported that working with patients was rewarding and felt overwhelmed because "patients are more acutely ill and complex and time pressures prevent good patient interactions" (Lemaire 2007). Thus, an important stressor for physicians is concern about their ability to provide optimal care for their patients (Wallace et al 2007).

According to Rick Hackett, professor of human resources management at McMaster University, "Exhaustion and illness in the workplace can lead to errors in judgment, difficulty in making decisions, increased social friction because of irritability and an increased risk of accidents due to decreased vigilance. Even more troubling is the potential for sick workers to spread illnesses" (Klie 2008).

Dr. Andrew Padmos, chief executive officer of the Royal College of Physicians and Surgeons of Canada, has stated that "At the foundation of everything we do is one simple aim: to provide the best possible health care for our patients." One result of this focus on patient safety has been the development of a *Safety Competencies Framework* in collaboration with the Canadian Patient Safety Institute. According to the framework, the six core domains shared by all health care professionals are to:

- contribute to a culture of patient safety,
- work in teams for patient safety,
- communicate effectively for patient safety,
- manage safety risks,
- optimize human and environmental factors, and
- recognize, respond to and disclose adverse events.

Generational and gender differences

Recent research shows that "baby-boomer" and "Gen-X" physicians work, on average, the same number of hours—61—per week and have a roughly equal level of commitment to patients. The biggest difference is that although Gen-Xers physicians feel that their medical careers are important, they "do not necessarily place [their work] at the forefront as the only aspect of who they are." However, the fact that the younger cohort seeks a well-rounded and balanced life can be interpreted by baby boomers as a lack of commitment (Jovic 2006).

The number of female physicians has increased 36.7 per cent since 1998 and they comprise 49.4 per cent of doctors under 40 (CIHI 2007).

In the 2007 National Physician Survey, 80 per cent of physicians indicated that the complexity of their patient caseload as the biggest factor affecting their time. Given an ever-increasing proportion of our aging population is affected by chronic disease and comorbidities, the average physician's workload will continue to grow (Rich 2008).

Work-life balance

Of the medical students who responded to the 2007 National Physician Survey, 60 per cent stated that the most important determinant of satisfaction and success in their medical practice is "the ability to achieve balance between work and personal life." (CFPC et al 2008). Younger physicians have indicated that they prefer to have good physical health rather than being stressed and tired out.

By emphasizing certain values in their work culture, physicians can help to mitigate the stressors that are part and parcel of their work. For example, discussions with "new" physicians highlight the value placed by this cohort on collegiality, open dialogue, mentorship and role modelling. Clear instructions during the orientation process help them to become more efficient and confident, translating into better teamwork and encouraging collegiality. Young physicians also express a desire for a positive work culture, along with a wish to avoid being drawn into any existing pockets of cynicism. They agree that any threat to their professional standards or that of a hospital is potentially stressful and can affect their relationship with patients. A culture of openness can help to mitigate these threats, and a healthy sense of community among the physicians can help physicians to cope with stressful situations.

Bill Wilkerson, co-founder of the Global Business and Economic Roundtable on Addiction and Mental Health, has noted: "You've got to understand the migratory sequence between stress, burnout and depression.

What is the solution in the workplace? Wilkerson puts it this way: "The solution is the cornerstone of good old-fashioned management, which is based on human decency, clear thinking, open communications. The other cornerstone is clarity of purpose and function."

Case resolution

The resident discussed with the program director family stresses combined with a heavy clinical workload which resulted in not being able to eat or sleep well and feeling burnout. The director recommended a visit to the family doctor for assessment. No physical or mental illness was detected. The family doctor recommended a balanced diet, exercise and spending time with family. The program director discussed the option of spending less time on extracurricular residency activities (work–life balance) and to ensure that preceptors are aware that residents should be excused from duties (e.g., following the post-call rules of the Poststaff Health Organization). One month later the resident is performing at their best and receives an excellent evaluation on their rotation. The resident also reports feeling better with respect to family relationships.

Key References

Canadian Medical Association. 2007. *Canadian Medical Association Launches First Check-up of Doctors' Health*. Ottawa: The CMA.

E. Societal expectations

Jordan Cohen, MD FRCPC

Objectives

This section will

- examine the challenge of balancing physician health with patients' expectations of their health care providers.

> ### Case
> A physician is ill and chooses to take a day off from his hospital-based practice. A number of patient visits are rescheduled, and students and residents are assigned to other supervisors. One of the rescheduled patients presents the following week but begins the clinical encounter by expressing dissatisfaction, anger and frustration that the postponement of the appointment resulted in losing extra time from work. The physician feels regretful and guilty at having taken the day off, but at the same time is frustrated by the patient's demanding tone.

Introduction

Society is quite aware of basic lifestyle choices that promote good health, such as maintaining a healthy diet, exercising regularly, avoiding smoking and street drugs, and limiting alcohol use. Most Canadians also recognize the importance of working with their primary care physician for health concerns, follow-up and appropriate screening at different stages of life. However, how often do patients consider the health needs of their own doctors?

Healthy physician, healthy patient

Some patients influence the mental health of their physicians by virtue of challenging personality traits, the denial of their own disease, over-dependence on their caregiver or intimidating interactions. Physicians may choose to prescribe unnecessary antibiotics for a viral illness to pacify the expectations of a patient who wants a quick resolution of their ailment. However, while these physicians are well aware of the lack of efficacy of antibiotics in these situations and the potential to promote new strains of resistant bacteria, they may feel they lack the time or energy to go through the process of proper patient education. The evolution of medicine into the computer era has also contributed to the complexity of the physician–patient relationship where physician health is concerned. Although one rarely hears of a house calls nowadays, e-mail is today's equivalent of yesterday's housecall. Patients can now follow doctors home, on vacation, or literally anywhere technology may go. Should doctors not be allowed to take time off, even from e-mail? What about the concept that patients need to be seen in person for a physician to make clinically informed decisions about their care? Today's society expects medicine to be a convenient service, similar to the fast-food industry—which likely contributed to the development of the walk-in clinic. However, the concept of easy access to non-urgent patient care may undermine even further a physician's ability to balance professional responsibilities with the self-care necessary to their own well-being. Society grants physicians status, respect, autonomy in practice, ability to self-regulate and financial compensation. In return, society has high expectations of physicians, including competence, altruism, ethical behaviour and the delivery of a high standard of care. Although in their professional role physicians must make their patients' well-being their first priority, this commitment must include a caveat for physician health. Physicians should bear in mind the advice given to airline passengers in case of a depressurization: put on one's own oxygen mask before assisting others. We must maintain our own health in order to be fit to care for society.

> ### Reflection for educators
> At the beginning of your residents' rotation, have them keep a journal of the challenges they encounter with respect to meeting the expectations of their patients and maintaining their own health. You may wish to provide your own example of challenges you have experienced. In addition, you can keep your own journal of such physician health challenges and have a formal discussion half-way through the rotation on how you and your residents dealt with your own challenges. At their regular evaluation meetings program directors can discuss with residents the process of dealing with these challenges. The journal will provide clear examples of how the residents understand the key issue. Residents may also consider incorporating such discussions into their half-day educational sessions or at their regular retreats.

Key references

Cruess SR, and RL Cruess. 2004. Professionalism and medicine's social contract with society. *Virtual Mentor*. 6 (4).

Gorlin R, Strain JJ, Rhodes R. 2001. Cultural collisions at the bedside: social expectations and value triage in medical practice. *Cambridge Quarterly of Healthcare Ethics*. 10 (1): 7–15.

Case resolution

The physician apologizes for the inconvenience the patient has experienced and explains that they were quite ill and possibly contagious. The patient appreciates the explanation and the frustration is alleviated.

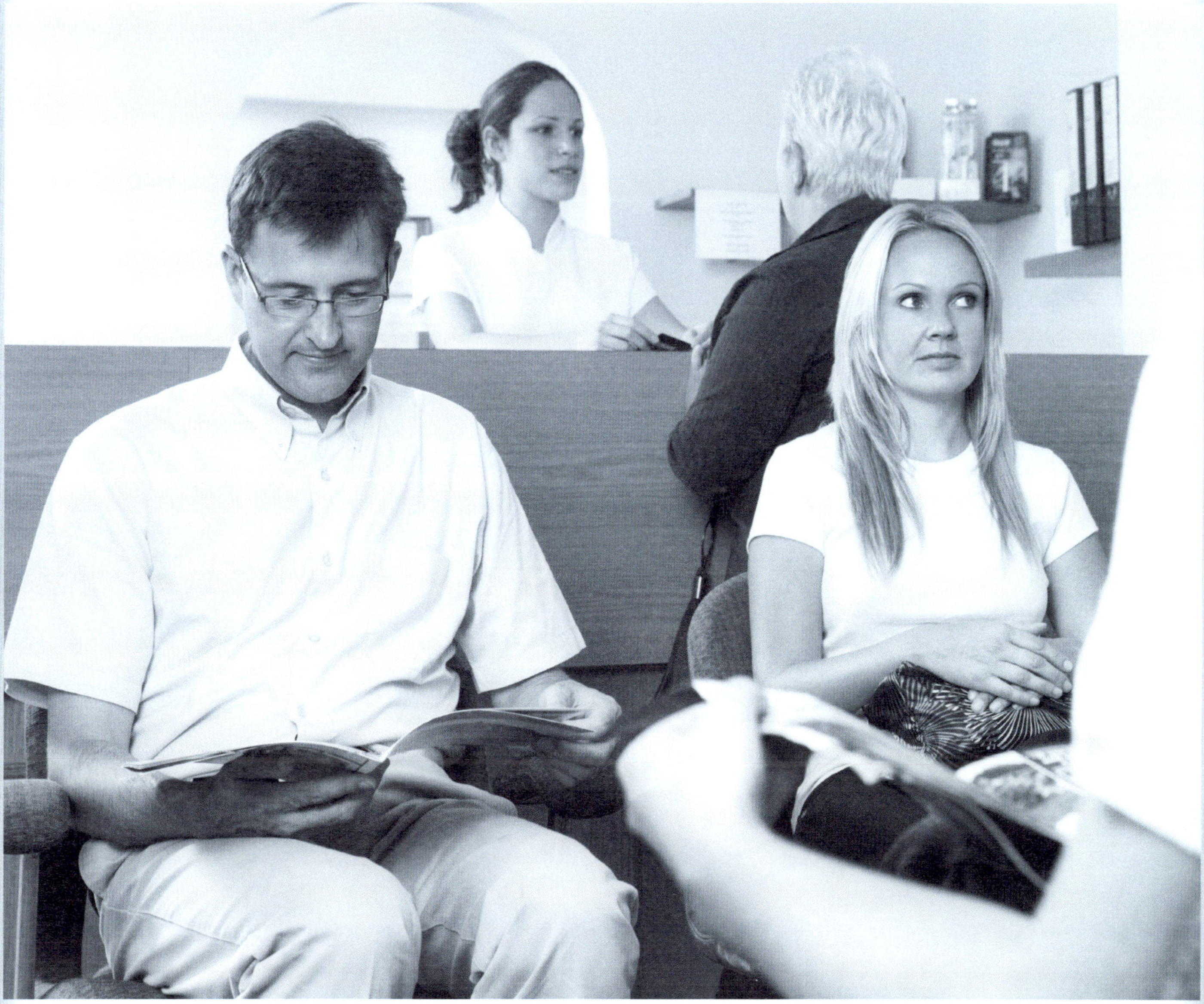

Introduction: The individual physician

Derek Puddester, MD MEd FRCPC

The CanMEDS Physician Health Guide is designed to be a reference tool that will allow readers to access specific information according to their personal needs. The chapters in this section acknowledge that individual physicians have an opportunity to identify and develop their skills in a several critical areas, namely personal awareness (described as values, beliefs and knowledge), reflective practice, emotional intelligence and leadership. Emerging evidence suggests that the development of skills in each of these areas is associated with improved personal health outcomes and professional sustainability.

Personal awareness

The vital importance of self-knowledge is the focus of the first chapter in this section. Starting with the perspective of Mahatma Gandhi, it considers what is meant by "values," "beliefs" and "knowledge." These building blocks of our world view influence every choice and decision we make and subtly guide us through our universe. Through exercises and reflection, readers will have an opportunity to consider how best they can become more aware of who they are and what they need to enjoy health and sustainability.

Reflective practice

Other professions and disciplines have long valued self-assessment, critical appraisal of the self, and introspection. This area is relatively new to medical training and practice, but other health professions have shown that reflective practice can enhance professional development, improve personal health, and promote patient care. The second chapter in this section introduces the basic principles of reflective practice, offering a simple model of reflective thinking and outlining the benefits of its implementation.

Emotional intelligence

The field of education has a rich history of influencing social development, cultural evolution and health outcomes. Referring to the work of thinkers such as Howard Gardiner, Peter Salovey, John Mayer and Daniel Goleman, the third chapter in this section suggests that models of emotional intelligence have much to offer the medical profession. Readers will be encouraged to consider several recommendations from the literature on emotional intelligence and will be challenged to assess and build on their strengths in this area.

Leadership

Outstanding leaders often achieve success by virtue of traits, characteristics and skills that they either possess innately or cultivate over time. Many of these elements can readily contribute to personal health and sustainability. Thus, in the last chapter of this section, readers are encouraged to consider practical suggestions to guide the development of their own leadership skills. A number of Canadian resources are identified that readers can readily access to enhance their understanding and practise of leadership.

There is no doubt that many other facets of health and sustainability are of relevance to physicians. Many other sections of *the CanMEDS Physician Health Guide* will be of value in your search for information and practical ways to move forward with your own personal health and professional sustainability strategy.

Key references

www.ephysicianhealth.com This free and anonymous online resource was written and designed by Canadian experts in physician health. Interactive and practical, it includes sections on relationships, depression and anxiety, resiliency, substance use, personal care and many other issues.

www.eworkplacehealth.com Also a free and anonymous online resource, this program focuses on the needs of health professionals in the workplace. Offering interactive exercises focused on the development of insight and skills, it blends many of the skills of this section of the guide and offers practical methods to enhance the health care workplace.

www.cma.ca The Canadian Medical Association's *Centre for Physician Health and Well-being* offers a rich clearinghouse of reference material on physician health, information on upcoming conferences and workshops, and additional learning resources on physician health.

A. The influence of values and beliefs on physician well-being

Derek Puddester, MD MEd FRCPC

Objectives

This chapter will

- discuss the influence of values and beliefs on physicians' health and well-being, and
- describe modes of self-reflection on personal health and wellness.

> **Case**
>
> A bright and clinically talented fellow has taken on many leadership roles and positions. One night, the fellow's spouse of four years asks for some time to talk. The fellow is shocked to learn that their spouse feels lonely in their marriage, feels disconnected, and is attracted to another person. The spouse asks for a period of separation so they can both consider how they want their marriage to move forward (or not).

Introduction

Your beliefs become your thoughts
Your thoughts become your words
Your words become your actions
Your actions become your habits
Your habits become your character
Your character becomes your destiny
Mahatma Gandhi

Physicians make hundreds of decisions every day. In general, these decisions are professional in nature and are shaped by years of training and experience. As physicians attain greater expertise, their clinical decisions can take on a more automatic character. Yet, as every medical student knows, if you ask a physician to explain their decision-making processes they can do so with clarity and confidence, and with reference to practical experience.

A physician's personal decisions are no different. Some decisions arise automatically on the basis of experience. This usually works well, but from time to time life throws us a curve ball, destabilizes us, and causes us to experience stress or even distress. At such times—indeed, at all times—it can be helpful to "check in" with our values and beliefs. This means being able to identify and define our core values, to explore and challenge our own belief systems, and to be open to new understanding. It also means being able to define where we are going by knowing where we have been.

Values

Values are complex, often abstract cognitive structures that shape our behaviour, give us motivation and drive, define our world view and help us determine what is important in life and what we appreciate in others. Some values seem universal to the human condition (love); others are culturally bound (universal health care). At the level of the individual, value systems arise primarily from familial circumstance and early life experience. For the most part, values are not open to change. They are deeply engrained, a core part of our identity, and central to our way of relating to the world. Debates based solely on values often result in a stalemate, as neither side, despite an exchange of perspectives and information is able to change.

> **Reflection**
>
> Identify six to eight roles that you have in your life at present (e.g., friend, child, parent, physician, lover, athlete) and list them. Then determine the proportion of your waking time that you dedicate to each of these roles. Rank your success in each role on a scale (0 = complete failure, 5 = average, 10 = complete success). Reflecting on the results, consider questions such as
>
> - Am I satisfied with these rankings?
> - Is there a link between each ranking and the time I spend in a given role?
> - Are there roles that I can let go of?
> - How could I reorganize my waking hours to dedicate more time to a particular role?
> - Are my expectations in line with those of others?
> - Should I share these rankings with my friends and family to see if they perceive things the same way?

It can be hard for people to identify their values, even though they act on them every day. Take the example of Susan, a busy oncologist early in her career. Because her parents travelled extensively for their work, she attended private boarding schools for most of her childhood and adolescence and did not have a close relationship with either parent. As an adult, she knows that she wants a different relationship with her children and husband, but this desire now appears to be in conflict with the demands of her new position as medical director of a large hospital-based program. Susan has become short-tempered and feels increasingly dissatisfied with her professional and personal roles. In speaking with a friend, she realizes that she is living life the way her parents did, and is deeply ashamed of her career choices. After reflecting on her core values, she resigns her administrative position and finds more time to spend with her family. And so her value conflict, although painful, proves to be useful in clarifying how she wants to spend her limited time and energy.

Beliefs

Beliefs are the cognitive structures we use to guide us through the world. Usually vague and unclear at the beginning, they are influenced by our family and friends. Increasingly, popular media and culture drive our beliefs, as does commercial industry. Our interface with the world serves to confirm or clarify our beliefs, which are generally somewhat in flux until they become solidified as "knowledge." Beliefs are usually malleable if we view new information as credible, reasonable and of value. This allows us to be open and flexible—traits that help us cope with new stressors and situations. At times, however, our beliefs can be so profoundly affirmed and validated that they become inflexible convictions. When rigid beliefs fail to help us in times of stress, we are faced with a challenge similar to value-based conflict. At other times, we might develop beliefs that are not based on fact or evidence (e.g., fantasies or assumptions); these too, can have a negative impact on our lives.

Beliefs that can be harmful include

- "I can control everything in my life."
- "It's not my fault."
- "If I don't talk about it then it doesn't exist."
- "I had no choice but to behave like that."
- "I'm always right."

The field of psychology has helped us appreciate the power of beliefs on health. Beliefs or "cognitions" have a powerful influence on our mood, our ability to initiate and maintain relationships, and our sense of self-worth. Sometime we entertain distorted beliefs that hold us back from achieving our goals and even from living our lives in line with our value systems. For example, physicians may be prone to "impostor syndrome," a distorted belief that they are not as competent as the world perceives them to be, that they are at constant risk of being "found out," and that they must put great effort into perfecting themselves. Some other, similarly damaging beliefs include:

- "I'm only as good a person as I am a physician."
- "Someday I'll get to slow down and enjoy life. This pace is temporary."
- "I am what I do. Being a physician means I'm a good person."
- "My family understands that work comes first."
- "My spouse understands that I'm tired when I come home."

Reflection

It isn't easy to request and accept feedback from other people. If the feedback isn't in keeping with our beliefs, it can precipitate a crisis of identity, security and confidence. By constantly and openly seeking feedback, or "checking in" with people who care about us, we can gain a better sense of what is actual and genuine.

Identify three or four people who love you and whom you trust. Let them know that you value them highly and respect their opinion. Then ask two or three questions, such as

- How is our relationship going? What do we do that is really great and what do we need to work on?
- How am I doing in my role as your [friend/partner/lover]? What do you like the most? What could I do better?
- How am I doing in balancing my professional role with my relationship with you? How do you think my life—my career being just one part it—is going right now? What are your top three pieces of advice?

Then give the person time to reflect and get back to you. When he or she does, listen very carefully. Avoid saying "but" or "maybe." Just listen. Say thank you and then reflect carefully on the comments. See how your beliefs are shaped by feedback. Explore the opportunities for growth. See if you can develop a routine of "checking in" with your friends and loved ones.

Case resolution

People often generalize their beliefs about themselves and others from one role to another. For example, feeling powerful and competent at work may be generalized into feelings of power and competence at home, even when others see things differently. Our sense of self is often stable and consistent across roles. Yet it is more likely that we have a variable sense of self in our roles, particularly roles that are new, novel or in flux.

The fellow likely generalized their sense of success from their professional life to their personal life, and seems to have believed that both situations were stable and successful. Although it is possible that the spouse withheld feedback purposely, it is also possible that neither chose to seek feedback or give it. As a result, the unhappiness came to light only when the spouse developed an attraction to another person, who represented, perhaps, what they felt was missing from the marriage.

Talking about feelings, identifying goals and sharing honest ideas and opinions helps to sustain spousal relationships. In the absence of sharing, assumptions will be created that might not be accurate. At this stage, the fellow and spouse should seek professional counselling to explore their immediate situation, determine if they want to maintain the relationship, and—if so—begin the process of repair and growth.

B. Reflective practice

Derek Puddester, MD MEd FRCPC

Objectives

This chapter will

- define reflective practice,
- suggest methods physicians can use to engage in reflective practice, and
- outline how reflective practice can promote individual health and wellness.

> **Case**
>
> During their first rotation, a resident observes a nurse slowly injecting an intravenous medication that ought to be pushed. The resident assumes the nurse knows better, as the nurse has more practice experience. The patient does not respond to the medication, and the resident repeats the order. Another nurse observes the error and yells out, "That's IV push!" The first nurse corrects the error, and the patient responds. The resident feels humiliated that they didn't raise a concern and spends the rest of the shift feeling stupid and weak.

What is reflective practice?

Many of us are creatures of habit. We learn, by observation or instruction, how we prefer to behave in particular types of situations. Over time, some behaviours become automatic, much like driving on a familiar street. But once in a while we encounter a different way of doing something that feels a bit better, or accept a tip from a friend or stranger. We adopt a new behaviour, and that too becomes automatic. Habits and routines bring stability and comfort.

The study and practise of medicine are no different. Physicians develop their preferred methods of interviewing patients, conducting physical examinations, breaking bad news and managing complications. These strategies become familiar, comfortable and routine.

When physicians find themselves facing personal or professional difficulties they, like all others, may benefit from a critical appraisal of established habits and routines. Reflective practice is a model of self-assessment and improvement that first emerged in the educational and social sciences literature. In recent decades it has been embraced by nursing and other health professions. It is only in recent years that it has caught the attention of medical educators and practitioners, leading to the development of a variety of strategies to help physicians critically appraise and potentially revise their methods of practice. The goal is to allow physicians to independently identify their strengths, limitations and vulnerabilities and, subsequently, areas for enhancement and development.

One benefit of reflective practice is that it improves the practitioner's ability to self-monitor and self-regulate performance; in turn, these skills contribute to the physician's overall resilience and to his or her ability to manage stress.

Stages of reflection

The reflective cycle proposed by Gibbs in 1988 comprises the following stages:

1. **Description:** What happened?
2. **Feelings:** What were you thinking and feeling during the event?
3. **Evaluation:** What was positive or negative about the event?
4. **Analysis:** How can you make sense of, or under stand, the event?
5. **Conclusions:** What alternatives to your action existed?
6. **Action plan:** What would you do the next time a similar event occurs?

There are different ways to apply the reflective cycle. Some find it helpful to use as a framework while engaged in a physical activity (e.g., working out at the gym, jogging, doing yoga) or in quiet meditation at the end of the day. Others require an active process such as painting, drawing, keeping a journal or composing music. Reflection can be exercised through a number of methods and media. Some physicians find it helpful to work through the reflective process in a group (the Balint method, which uses guided small-group case discussions to examine the physician–patient relationship, often uses a form of reflective cycle) or with a mentor or colleague. Chapter 2-D of this handbook introduces the "personal board of directors" concept—a useful tool in promoting one's ability to reflect on practice.

Other benefits of reflective practice

A reflective stance is empowering. It allows the practitioner to take ownership of clinical experiences that might otherwise be frustrating or draining. In addition, reflection on established and comfortable ways of learning and practising can push the physician in new directions, facilitating personal and professional growth and development, enhancing clinical skills and improving outcomes. Also, by being open to feedback, reflective practice encourages flexibility in the face of stress and change, which in turn helps others to feel comfortable with the practitioner and his or her style.

Reflective practice should not be pursued excessively. A few minutes each day or dedicated time a few times a week is all that it takes for the constructive reflection that can enhance health and wellness. By working through the cycle using a recent, typical event (e.g., being asked to stay late post-call, deciding to skip lunch to get dictations done, choosing to study instead of going to the gym) physician learners can discover some strategies to enhance their health and well-being with relative ease.

Case resolution

The resident meets with their mentor, who walks through the reflective cycle. The resident realizes they were feeling inexperienced and apprehensive during the event. The resident knew what was required, which was positive, but did not engage appropriately with the team to ensure that it was delivered correctly. The resident realizes the need to work on team skills, including assertiveness and being comfortable in the new role as a licensed physician. When a similar event occurs a few months later the resident quietly states, "IV push, please." This facilitates appropriate patient care as well as enhancing the resident's personal and professional confidence.

Key references

Epstein R. 1999. Mindful practice. *Journal of the American Medical Association*. 282: 833–9.

Gibbs G. 1988. *Learning by Doing: A Guide to Teaching and Learning Methods*. Oxford: Further Education Unit, Oxford Polytechnic.

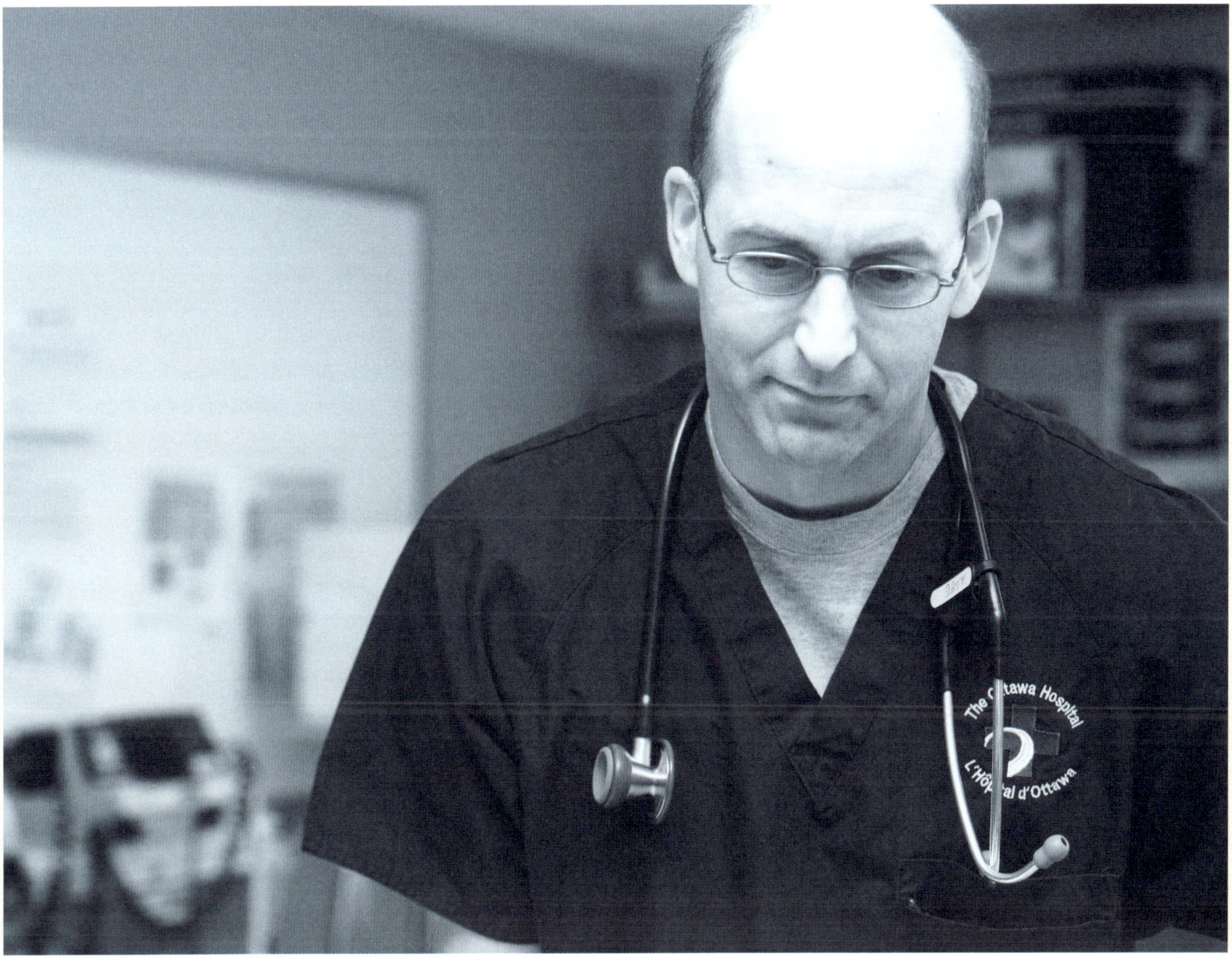

C. Emotional intelligence

Derek Puddester, MD MEd FRCPC

Objectives

This chapter will

- describe emotional intelligence and several of its components,
- outline ways in which physicians can develop their own emotional intelligence, and
- illustrate how emotional intelligence can promote individual health and group collegiality.

> **Case**
>
> A first-year resident quickly masters whatever is read and readily acquires new skills. However, the resident has a reputation among their peers for being narcissistic, domineering and self-promoting. The resident is not particularly involved with classmates and is not an especially popular member of the care team. Although no one has given direct feedback on this interpersonal style, the resident is aware that they have few friends, no intimate relationships, and little connection to others. The resident is uncertain how to manage things differently.

What is emotional intelligence?

A long-standing and almost exclusive reliance on standardized IQ testing to assess individuals' intelligence began to shift profoundly in the early 1990s with the publication of psychologist Howard Gardner's *Frames of Mind,* a landmark text that introduced evidence to support his theory that people have multiple forms of intelligence: linguistic, logical-mathematical, musical, spatial, bodily-kinesthetic, interpersonal, intrapersonal and (a later addition) naturalist. Gardner noted that once learners' innate intelligences were identified, teachers could design appropriate educational strategies to facilitate their learning. For example, linguistic learners would learn mainly by word-based exercises, visual cues and pictures would help spatial learners, and social experiences would help interpersonal learners.

About a decade later, further work by psychologists Peter Salovey and John Mayer on emotional intelligence was popularized by a New York Times science writer, Daniel Goleman, who described emotional intelligence in terms of a framework based on the five elements described below.

Self-awareness. People with emotional intelligence have insight into their talents and vulnerabilities and seek ways to improve and develop. They understand their own emotions and those felt by others.

Self-regulation. Emotional impulses can be compelling; those with high emotional intelligence regulate these impulses and avoid making impulsive decisions. They cope well in the face of change and have a remarkable flexibility and adaptability. Finally, they are able to manage tasks well and avoid becoming overcommitted or stretched too thin.

Motivation. Emotionally intelligent people are focused, hard-working, productive and welcome a challenge. They tend to be "finishers" who complete tasks fully. They keep their eye on the goal and defer immediate gratification.

Empathy. Emotionally intelligent people recognize and appreciate the emotional needs and wants of others and are able to communicate this understanding to others honestly and openly. This helps them to develop many excellent relationships; they are known as active and thoughtful listeners—as "real" people.

Social skills. Identified as team players, emotionally intelligent people focus on the success of those around them, are outstanding communicators, and are skilled at maintaining healthy relationships. They also are aware when relationships are not particularly healthy and are skilled at disengaging from such relationships or keeping them at an appropriate distance.

In summary, emotionally intelligent people are warm and engaging, comfortable and safe to be around, easy to connect with and collaborate with, and generally cheerful and energizing. They are social success stories and enjoy positive personal and professional outcomes.

Promoting one's own emotional intelligence

Emotional intelligence is valuable for a number of reasons, but of particular importance is the insight it affords into one's own feelings and behaviours, thus promoting a more genuine approach to life and practice. The literature on this subject area offers a range of recommendations on cultivating one's emotional intelligence. Key points are summarized here with the needs of medical residents particularly in mind. Attending workshops and lectures can also be an efficient way to learn strategies to enhance emotional intelligence.

Physician, know thyself. This is all about digging deep: knowing why you wanted to be a physician in the first place, why you make the choices you do in friendships and relationships, why you react to patients, peers and supervisors the way you do, understanding parts of yourself that you don't like (or that others don't like), seeing if you want or need to make any changes, and knowing where you want to go in life and in your career. Be prepared for the occasional unpleasant surprise. As you go through residency and training you will face new and unique challenges, and you might not always be prepared for the way you react.

Assess and develop your emotional literacy. Emotional literacy refers to skill in perceiving and expressing feelings. A simple starting-point in building emotional literacy can be to practise using three-word sentences such as "I feel happy" or "I feel scared." Avoid "blaming" sentences that begin with "You" (e.g., "You're too bossy," as opposed to "I feel excluded from your decisions."). Practise grading feelings and emotions using a 1–10 scale, and learn adjectives that help communicate your understanding (e.g., "You seem distraught").

Communicate feelings clearly. This can be a challenge, since many of us are socialized to suppress our emotions. Our feelings and our body language are often mismatched (e.g., smiling in displeasure or frustration); we tend to use a small range of words to describe feelings, thus missing opportunities to accurately describe what we observe (e.g., everything is "fantastic" or "sad" with nothing in between); and we might project the same response (e.g., skepticism, dominance, blunt neutrality) no matter what the situation, leading others to wonder about our true feelings. Unless doing so would be harmful, it is best to take full ownership of our feelings and to communicate them genuinely and directly.

Develop insight into your negative feelings. Such feelings are often expressions of unmet emotional needs. Although people have a diverse range of needs, some that are frequently unmet include being accepted, appreciated, heard, included, loved, needed, respected, safe and valued. Needs are powerful drivers of behaviour. Unsatisfied needs can lead people to act in unconstructive ways. For example, not feeling loved or accepted could be managed by seeking close friendships, joining team sports or clubs, or developing a skill or talent. Alternatively, one could control or manipulate others into loving and accepting them, or become excessively competitive, narcissistic or self-promoting.

Take ownership of your emotions. People often avoid taking responsibility for their feelings, particularly when they are unpleasant. This is often where people's defences become activated and relationships start to fail. When you feel unpleasant emotions, take full ownership of them by using "I statements" to describe your feelings (e.g., "I felt really scared that my patient would die and it would be my fault," as opposed to "That stupid nurse didn't give me the blood work in time and the patient could have died."). It is also important to "own up" to actions that hurt others and to try to make them right (e.g., "I'm sorry if I was condescending. The truth is that I'm exhausted and I wasn't paying attention to my body language. It doesn't make it right, I know it upset you, and I am honestly sorry about that."). Examine closely how you cope with stress and how your style affects others: are you a team player, or do you focus mainly on yourself and express your stress by whining, complaining or dominating others?

Examine your sense of teamwork. Residency is a time of incredible personal and professional demands. In general, if you are skilled at working in and for teams, residency will be successful. People will watch your back and you will watch theirs. If you react to stress by becoming insular, you may be putting your health and well-being at risk. Try to stay connected to others, support and nurture the relationships that emerge during residency, and get involved with your residency program and its various activities. It's okay to focus on your own career ambitions, too, but not at the expense of others. By helping your peers to shine, you'll develop your own leadership skills and your emotional intelligence.

Case resolution

The resident attends a weekend workshop on emotional intelligence and realizes that they had many unmet emotional needs from both the present and the past. The resident begins to pay closer attention to the needs of colleagues and works on active listening and empathy. The resident soon notices that others warm to this approach and compliment the resident on the "different approach." The resident strives to be cheerful and positive and volunteers to help with the resident retreat. The resident also begins to work with a coach to develop better insight into emotional issues. Over time, the resident begins to appreciate the importance of emotions in their own life and the lives of others. The sense of isolation dissipates, and feelings of depression lift.

Key references

Gardner H. 1993. *Frames of Mind.* New York: Basic Books.

Goleman D. 2006. *Emotional Intelligence.* 10th anniversary edition. New York: Bantam Books.

D. Leadership and leadership skills

Derek Puddester, MD MEd FRCPC

Objectives

This chapter will

- consider the meaning of leadership from a personal and professional perspective,
- suggest ways in which physicians can develop their leadership skills, and
- describe how leadership skills can help promote personal and professional health and wellness.

> **Case**
>
> In the final year of a fellowship a physician wonders if there will be a job available when they are done. The fellowship has been a rewarding experience, and the physician feels confident in their skills and knowledge. But the fellow's supervisors seem to be buckling under the strain of the system, morale seems to be at an all-time low, and the word on the street is that the future is bleak. Usually a cheerful and positive person, the physician is starting to feel a little scared. Has all of this work been for nothing?

Introduction

Much has been written about leadership and how it influences us as individuals and as a society. Many of us need leaders to give us a sense of direction, stability, purpose and hope. Others do not grativate toward leaders, maintaining their identity more autonomously. And then there are those who thrive by leading.

In general, leaders are average people who differ from their peers in some ways and mirror them in others. These are people who were born with an innate set of talents and skills (not as common as one might think) and or who grew to develop such a portfolio over time. Regardless of their nature or nurture, leaders have a clear sense of their values and beliefs, have the social skills to attract and maintain relationships with others in a way that motivates action on those values and beliefs, and maintain a transparency, integrity and genuineness that foster the trust of those who choose to follow.

How do you become a leader?

Leadership can be demonstrated in any sphere of action, and on any scale, to bring about positive change and promote improved outcomes. For residents, the acquisition of leadership skills is an important aspect of their development as medical professionals. The following discussion explores a set of catch-phrases that can inspire the cultivation of leadership skills among new physicians.

Get involved. Many organizations could use your energy, ideas and vision. Your program and its host university will have committees that welcome, and need, resident input; your provincial housestaff organization (PHO) is managed and led by residents and would welcome your input with open and grateful arms; your provincial medical association welcomes and needs resident input; and your national organizations (Canadian Association of Interns and Residents, Canadian Medical Association, Royal College of Physicians and Surgeons of Canada, Canadian Association for Medical Education, and your specialty society) have roles and purposes for resident input. You can also partner with international development agencies to offer your skills abroad, or consider working with Medécins Sans Frontières after graduation. All of these organizations offer opportunities to put your ideas and personality to the test with lots of support, encouragement and, in many cases, formal training.

Many organizations outside of medicine would also welcome your input and energy. Habitat for Humanity, Big Brothers/Big Sisters, the United Way, political parties and non-governmental organizations also present opportunities for leadership development and for personal and professional growth.

Get passionate. Reflect for a while on your core values and beliefs: What it is that most creates energy or tension within you? Perhaps you are a passionate defender of socialized medicine. Perhaps you are a proponent of greater privatization. Perhaps you have a new idea that merits attention. Seek out the people and organizations who would appreciate your contribution and leadership. If a cause puts fire in your belly, it will sustain your ability to lead. And so, identify your passions and get busy.

Get goal-oriented. Spreading yourself too thin will produce mediocre results. Pick one or two areas of leadership and apply yourself to them as best you can. Not only will this help you maintain balance in your life, it will also help you succeed in those things that you choose to take on. Be a finisher. Leaders didn't get to where they are by stopping half-way down the track.

Get honest and real. Get to know yourself really well. Most leaders can readily identify their critical strengths as perceived by themselves and others. They can also readily identify their vulnerabilities, flaws and shortcomings—again, as perceived by themselves and others. Be yourself and be genuine: superficiality and phoniness are easy for others to detect. Learn to be comfortable in your own skin, how to use your own strengths and talents, and how to adapt your style of interpersonal engagement to meet the needs of others and the situation at hand.

Get trained. Leadership skills develop over time. Most successful leaders have had the benefit of some form of formal leadership training. Typically, leadership courses offer assessment of personality traits and interpersonal styles as part of their curriculum. This process, although sometimes a little painful, is well worth the investment of time and course fees. Ask your provincial or national housestaff and medical associations for their recommendations for leadership training, and also consider opportunities such as the Royal College's *Annual Resident Leadership Program* and the CMA's *Physician-Manager Institute.* You can also encourage your program director to develop a local leadership program as part of the core curriculum.

Get ready to learn from mistakes. As you develop leadership skills you will make mistakes. Despite your best intentions, you will bruise feelings, leave people out, subvert processes, create unintentional consequences and perhaps even do harm. Seek lots of feedback on your leadership efforts, learn the techniques of reflective practice, and develop a process of modifying your own leadership strategies as you move forward.

Get a board of directors. Leaders identify mentorship as one of the critical elements of a successful career. Everyone benefits from mentorship and by mentoring others. In general, mentors are individuals that negotiate a relationship that focuses primarily on the growth and development of the less experienced of the pair, and some mentors actively seek ways to promote the career development of their mentee. These relationships can be incredibly satisfying and often last for many years. Indeed, some people have a number of mentors, each of whom helps with a particular area of development (e.g., one for clinical research, one for leadership, one for educational development, one for grant writing, etc.). This collection of experts can be your personal "board of directors" and can enrich your career and life development.

Get the link between leadership and physician health. Leadership development is a tremendous opportunity to focus on your own resiliency. The insights gained in leadership development, particularly with respect to identifying your core values and beliefs, your interpersonal style and your personality traits, are powerful and practical. When things are stressful and difficult, and your vulnerabilities become apparent, your leadership skills and traits can help you to cope well. In addition, your leadership skills can help promote a system of medicine that promotes the health and well-being of all involved, including all health professionals as well as the patients and families they serve.

Summary

Specialty medicine has embraced the belief that it has much to offer in the leadership of health, health care, medical training and education, medical research and medical politics. The Royal College, particularly through its CanMEDS Framework, stresses that leadership is an important role for the specialist physician and is encouraging trainees to acquire a broad array of skills that will cultivate their leadership ability. An added benefit of leadership development is that it often contributes to personal health and well-being and enhances physician sustainability.

Case resolution

The fellow asks to meet with the chief and is surprised to discover that they have very similar concerns. The chief asks the fellow to join two teams: a working group that is completing an informal review of the department, and a national task force focused on physician resources. The fellow feels that the personal investment of time and energy will be worthwhile, and so also signs up for a local leadership program. Over the course of the next year, the fellow makes a number of helpful contacts, one of whom agrees to be their mentor. With their support, the fellow finds an excellent position in a neighbouring province. The fellow keeps in touch with their former program director and is pleased to learn that a number of the recommendations from the informal review have been implemented and are successful.

Key references

Collins-Nakai R. 2006. Leadership in medicine. *McGill Journal of Medicine.* 9: 68–73.

Dowton SB. 2004 Leadership in medicine: Where are the leaders? *Medical Journal of Australia* 181: 652–54.

Introduction: Balancing personal and professional life

Jordan Cohen, MD FRCPC

Many physicians enjoy high levels of satisfaction at work and in their family lives. However, establishing and maintaining a healthy equilibrium between professional and personal life is not easy, and it is not uncommon for practising physicians and residents to struggle with time management, competing demands between work and home, and tensions in intimate relationships. Physicians' work-life balance is shaped by many factors, including workload, practice specialty and setting, the availability of mentors, sleep patterns, personality traits and challenging scenarios (e.g., death, suffering, medical errors, malpractice suits). However, perhaps the strongest determinant of a healthy work-life balance is the ability to control one's schedule and the total number of hours worked.

Canadian surveys have shown that most physicians believe their workload is too heavy and that their family and personal lives have suffered because of their choice of medicine as a career. A lack of balance between work and home life can lead to psychological distress and even burnout. On the job, the consequences may include cynicism, decreased job satisfaction, poor work performance and absenteeism. These stresses can spill over into personal life, straining relationships and leading to family discord and isolation from friends.

The Canadian Medical Association's *Policy on Physician Health and Well-being* emphasizes that physicians should be aware of the essential components of well-being, such as rest, exercise, healthy nutrition and a happy family life. The Royal College of Physicians and Surgeons of Canada have stressed the importance of professional sustainability as a key competency under the CanMEDS Professional Role. Geurts and associates, researched how the association between residency training and home life interface on the psychological well-being of medical residents. They identified four risk factors for a disrupted work–home balance: having a spouse who works overtime often, an unfavourable work schedule, a large workload and a poor relationship with one's superior.

If physicians lead by example by discussing their own positive lifestyle habits, this might even motivate their patients to adopt similarly healthy behaviours. Thus, an argument can be made that medical education should encourage health professionals to practise and exhibit healthy lifestyles. Recommendations have been made on the basis of research findings that spending more personal time with friends and family can decrease stress.

In an effort to promote physician health and wellness, doctors must ensure that they have their own family physician, be alert to colleagues in need of support, and when appropriate initiate appropriate methods of intervention, including referrals to physician health programs. For the professional culture of medicine to achieve a healthy balance between work and home life, these concepts must not only be taught, but must also be strongly encouraged by individuals in positions of authority at all levels of medical education.

The following chapters will discuss how to maintain positive interpersonal relationships during training and throughout one's career. Specific attention will be paid to physicians' relationships with their spouses and their children.

Key references

Armstrong A, Alvero R, Dunlow S, Nace M, Baker V, Stewart E. 2009. Balancing the professional and personal. *Journal of Fertility and Sterility*. 91 (1): 18–21.

Canadian Medical Association. 1998. *Physician Health and Well-being* [policy]. Ottawa: The CMA.

Geurts S, Rutte C, Peeters M. 1999. Antecedents and consequences of work-home interference among medical residents. *Social Science & Medicine*. 48 (9): 1135–48.

A. Maintaining relationships during training and beyond

Jordan Cohen, MD FRCPC

Objectives

This chapter will

- list common problems in personal relationships experienced by medical trainees, and
- describe some interventions that can improve the personal relationships of physicians.

> **Case**
>
> The program director of a mid- to large-sized residency program is facing a challenge. Most of the residents in the program have intimate partners, and several have children. One of the residents told the program director that this resident had not had a chance to spend meaningful time with their partner, with the exception of a yearly vacation. They were unhappy with this, and considering switching programs.

Introduction

Certain traits that seem to go with the territory of medicine can have a detrimental effect on physicians' personal lives. An exaggerated sense of responsibility, guilt and self-doubt, perfectionism, a desire for control, and a drive to overwork can lead to self-neglect and the derailment of intimate relationships. Warde and colleagues, reported increased marital and parental satisfaction have been closely associated with a decrease in conflict between professional and familial roles. Minimizing the conflict between the demands training and home-life, and having a supportive partner are considered important factors in both parental and marital satisfaction.

When physicians neglect their own care, always need to be in control, use work as an escape from personal life and do not define appropriate boundaries between work and home life, they set themselves up for relationship problems. In addition, many doctors are embarrassed to find that they need relationship help. They are often "wounded healers" who have already faced stressors that make them vulnerable to mental illness, or who have undiagnosed mental health problems (e.g., mood disorders and substance dependence). One can imagine that such problems are likely to be compounded in spousal relationships in which both partners are physicians. Although the onset of relationship difficulties can be insidious, physicians should be alert to the warning signs, such as more frequent or intense arguments, increased drinking, excessive immersion in work, decreased physical intimacy, or simply an inability to communicate one's feelings to one's partner. Useful strategies that develop and safeguard intimacy in a relationship include: protecting time to communicate with one's partner; reading about the dynamics of relationships; attending a marital retreat; attending couples therapy; and taking time to manage one's own health needs (e.g., through regular appointments with a family physician).

> **Reflection for educators**
>
> Get to know the spouses and significant others in the lives of the residents in your program early on in residency training. Educate residents' spouses about the physician health resources available to their families (e.g., physician health programs). These individuals are often the first to recognize problems in their physician spouses and in their family relationships.

Many workplace interventions can help to reduce the toll taken on physicians' personal lives. Adequate vacation time, flexible work hours and equitable part-time work are conditions of employment that are conducive not only to improved family life and mental well-being but also to greater job satisfaction and productivity. Physicians are most satisfied as parents when they have a supportive spouse and when the work–home conflicts of both partners are minimal. The location and type of medical practice can also affect physicians' relationships with their children. For instance, Armstrong's group, found that physicians who worked for a salary were more fulfilled in their parental role than physicians who worked on fee-for-service basis. Finally, the employment status of one's spouse seems to play a role in parental satisfaction. Physicians with spouses who were professionals and/or stay-at-home parents had a higher level of parental satisfaction.

Case resolution

The program director organizes a day-long retreat for the residents and their significant others. The program director brings in a well-known speaker to discuss issues surrounding physician health, including work-lifebalance, ways to maintain healthy intimate relationships, and recognizing mental health problems. The resident body finds the experience very useful and decide to make this an annual event to help prevent family stress related to residency training and to help recognize the roles that each of their families play in their own residency program.

Key references

Myers MF. 2004. Medical marriages and other intimate relationships. *Medical Journal of Australia.* 181 (7): 392–4.

Warde CM, Moonesinghe K, Allen W, Gelberg L. 1999. Marital and parental satisfaction of married physicians with children. *Journal of General Internal Medicine.* 14: 157–65.

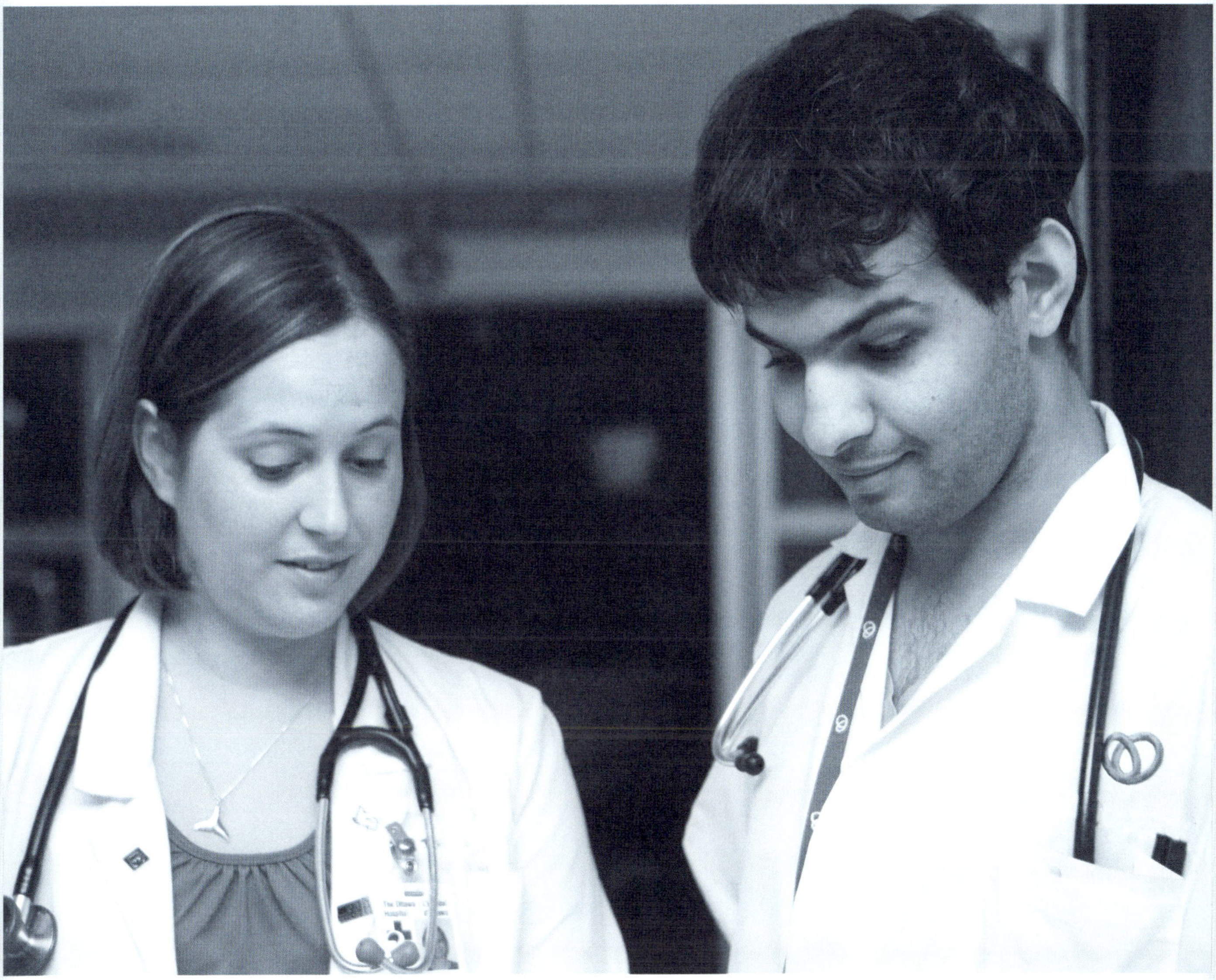

B. Promoting healthy partnerships in medical families

Dianne Maier, MD FRCPC

Objectives

This chapter will

- discuss the importance of healthy spousal relationships in medical families, and
- explore challenges specific to those relationships.

> **Case**
>
> A resident requests a meeting with their supervisor over coffee. The resident becomes distraught while disclosing that she miscarried her first pregnancy three weeks ago and that her partner, a more senior resident, is preoccupied with preparing for a fellowship position in another city. The resident acknowledges that her partner has tried to be supportive, but feels that "he just doesn't get it." Her colleagues remain unaware of her pregnancy and loss, and she is fearful of them knowing anything.

Introduction

Successful marriages and similar partnerships are built on knowledge, friendship, fondness and admiration (Gottman 1999). For physicians as for anyone else, this means having time together to develop the essential advantage of such relationships: intimacy. Intimacy means connection, identification as a couple, trust and a sense of mutuality. It includes affection, expressiveness, sexuality, cohesion, compatibility, autonomy and conflict resolution (Myers 2001).

Work and family life

The issue of deferring intimacy in favour of medical work has been described in the literature on medical marriages (Myers 2001 and Gabbard 1989). Some physicians choose professional advancement over the nurturing of intimate relationships, working long hours at the expense of their home lives. Physicians' family relationships suffer when they chronically postpone their investment in the "emotional bank account" of their families or in some cases, avoid admitting that they in fact prefer work to family life. Paradoxically, however, "the marital relationship is the main source of coping with the stress of medical practice" (Gabbard 1989).

Physicians who enjoy successful intimate partnerships learn early that certain attributes that serve them well at work are counterproductive at home. For example, while physicians are accustomed to their role as experts and expect to be in control, their partners should not "take orders" and require an equal influence in family life (Gottman 1999). In contrast to most physicians' experience of medical education, marriage is non-competitive. Nor is perfection required or even desirable. Relationships, however, do require work in realtime, a sense of humour, and a degree of luck. John Gottman, a respected researcher in marriage and relationships, stresses the importance of positive sentiment in successful marriages. When mutually positive sentiment overrides negative sentiment from day to day, couples can acknowledge one another in a non-judgmental and supportive way and enjoy true partnership. It is also important to value the work and other pursuits of one's partner, inside and outside the home, whether medical or not.

As seductive as the practise of medicine can be, Michael Myers reminds us to "say yes to the relationship and practise saying no to other offers" (Myers 2001). Spend a minimum of twenty minutes alone with your spouse each day and plan a date together every week.

Monica Hill and Nancy Love quote the novelist Henry James in their workshops on physicians' relationships: "Three things in human life are important. The first is to be kind. The second is to be kind. The third is to be kind." Within the circle of kindness, each partner has responsibility to work toward the resolution of conflict. Unbalanced criticism, defensiveness, ridicule, a posture of superiority, and "shutting off" are poisonous to this process (Hill and Love 2008). As in the general population, domestic violence and abuse occurs in medical families too. It is unacceptable and a response of appropriate professional assistance is important.

Dual-physician relationships

Conflict between work and familial roles is inevitable at times, whether one or both partners are physicians. Classically, role strain has been more frequently noted among female physicians, but in reality male physicians experience it as well. Half of married women physicians are married to other physicians (Sobecks et al 1999). Dual-physician relationships bring certain challenges, such as complicated schedules and career compromises, even when the compromise is an alleged "one time only" career opportunity (Schrager et al 2007). Careers can be shaped, reshaped and salvaged more easily than relationships and families. On the other hand, sharing professional interests can be satisfying, which can lead to greater mutual understanding, support and shared parenting (Schrager et al 2007). It would seem, however, whether by preference, mutual decision or default, that women physicians continue to take more responsibility on the home front than their male counterparts. A new trend may also be emerging with higher numbers of female physicians being the primary or sole income earner in their households.

Protecting and nurturing our intimate relationships may require a re-examination of our professional responsibilities and work environment. As you develop your resident group or consider your eventual practice setting, keep these questions in mind:

- Does your group discuss shock-absorber systems for parental leaves and urgent family issues? Does it have

flexible work plans? How does it deal with illness, sabbaticals and career transitions?
- Are all generations of physicians involved?
- Has someone led the way?
- What is the group's experience with dual medical career families? (Rubin 2006).

It is also important to plan with regard to that important geographical triangle: home, school and workplace. Keeping logistics as simple as possible will benefit your marriage and family in the long run.

Raising children together

For many women physicians, the question of when to plan childbearing is especially challenging when training demands and biological clocks collide (Straehley 2006). Supportive colleagues and training programs are nearly as important as a supportive partner. A physician mother never forgets how she was treated by colleagues during pregnancy. Furthermore, residency training directors never accompany graduated residents to the infertility clinic.

The concept that it takes a village to raise a child applies to medical families, too. Women physicians are particularly aware that the more they work, and the greater number of children they choose to have, the greater the chance that they will need to rely on child care arrangements beyond the family. Many women physicians and dual-career couples find live-in help with regard to child care invaluable. External assistance with regard to other household duties can also be a time-management tool that benefits everyone.

Two points to remember when your medical relationship is blessed with children are these:

1. You do not have to be perfect, but you can be good enough.
2. "The lives of children do not wait" (Warde 1996).

Although little has been written about the children of physicians, we do know that children want and deserve their parents' time and attention. Depending on their stage of development, this may mean breastfeeding for the recommended time, taking the maximum possible parental leave, delaying a career move, or signing out to a colleague more often. Even if you cannot always be there, it is important to work with your partner and to communicate with your child so that you are emotionally involved and up-to-date with what is going on in your child's life (Sotile and Sotile 2000).

Managing work and family time

It is important to reflect on the impact of on-call commitments on our partners, whether or not they are also physicians, and on our children. Many of us display mood and behavioural changes in anticipation of on-call duty and when we return home post-call. When taking a call from home, consider the impact on your family, whose sleep is being disturbed by the phone or by your departure to the hospital (Maier 2005). Enlist your partner in your fatigue management plan.

Case resolution

At the supervisor's suggestion, the resident and her partner access couples counselling and discuss what the pregnancy had meant to them. She is concerned about her biological clock and that she and her spouse have delayed their family, and other aspects of life together, long enough. She had speculated that a child would keep her relationship together, given her partner's attraction to "more medicine" and achievement. In further marital sessions she understands that her partner's grief is different but as valid as her own. He expresses fear of giving in to his feelings lest they derail his career focus. With the counsellor's help, they review their priorities with regard to career plans and the timing of child-bearing. These sessions lead to a better understanding of their mutual objectives, and of the supports available to them to help them meet their goals.

Vacations are one of the non-urgent but important elements of time management. Vacations in which play and fun—and not perfection—are modelled, where being rather than doing are valued and pleasure for its own sake is enjoyed, are healthy for the whole family (Maier 2005)

Summary

Managing the expectations of our partners and others can be problematic in medical relationships. Some of these expectations may be financial, arising from assumptions about what the lifestyles of physicians will be. Some may involve an expectation of concierge service within the health care system. And some may simply relate to being sandwiched between our children and our parents as we reach midlife. Expectations in any of these areas can lead to relationship stress. All deserve reflection, good communication and attention to maintaining appropriate and ubiquitous boundaries.

Relationships go through cycles. Should your medical marriage run into challenges, remember you are not alone. Dr. Michael Myers, through his book *Doctors' Marriages*, shares his wisdom that face-to-face couples' therapy works best. Seek professional help through your community resources or your physician health program. Getting help is a sign of strength, and a sign of commitment to your relationship.

Key references

Myers MF. 2001. The well-being of physician relationships. *Western Journal of Medicine*. 174: 30–3.

Sotile WM and MO Sotile. 2000. *The Medical Marriage*. Chicago: American Medical Association.

C. Physician parents: Unique issues

Leah J. Dickstein, MD MA DLFAPA and Derek Puddester, MD MEd FRCPC

Objectives

This chapter will

- describe some of the challenges commonly faced by physician parents,
- summarize supports that programs can use to facilitate sustainability of residents who are parents, and
- identify strategies for resident physicians to promote their own development as parents.

> **Case**
>
> A second-year resident has recently adopted an infant with their partner. In general, they are surrounded by love and support. However, several residents in the year are off on parental leave, and the frequency of call is higher than usual. Several colleagues mention that they hope the resident is not planning on taking parental leave, as that would increase call frequency to 1:4. In fact, the resident is planning on taking leave, but is now dreading approaching the program director with a request.

Introduction

Great joy comes with being a parent. Children add a dimension to life that is unique and delightful, and the parental role provides opportunities to know ourselves better. That being said, parenting can add to the complexity of managing busy personal and professional lives. Where some may argue that physician parents lack full professional commitment, others may perceive that physicians lack parental selflessness. Issues confronting physician parents are many, and their complexities concern both professional and personal roles.

Parental leave

Every provincial housestaff organization has negotiated parental leave policies for their members, and many directly address leaves for both biological and adopted children. These policies mesh nicely with the principles and goals of the federal parental leave program and allow many trainees up to a year of leave. Residents should be supported and, indeed, encouraged to take advantage of parental leave during their training. Healthy attachment and bonding with a child requires time. Adequate leave also allows for the entire family to grow together as they move through the phases of expectation, arrival, integration and, finally, resumption of professional roles. An investment in physician families is a smart one and directly contributes to the long-term sustainability of the physician workforce.

Career choices

Specialty medicine in Canada is experiencing significant demographic shifts, including with respect to the gender and age of practitioners. More women than ever before are practising in the specialties, including areas that traditionally were male dominated. In addition, more men than ever before are taking advantage of parental leave policies. Thus, traditional gender roles in Canadian culture are clearly undergoing a healthy evolution. However, these shifts have created new challenges for training programs as they strive to balance principles of sound education and training, human rights and responsibilities, and health care human resource issues. This juggle can be difficult and often requires innovation, flexibility and creativity. Medical students are watching this transition and may choose not to engage in specialty medicine if it is perceived to be adverse to their family-related values and expectations.

In the meantime, academic medicine has not been particularly kind to physician parents who have typically enjoyed less institutional support (research funding, mentorship, administrative support) than non-parents, tend to have fewer publications, perceive a slower progression of career goals, and have lower levels of career satisfaction. For academic specialty medicine to remain robustly grounded in scholarship, new mechanisms of career and professional development need to be explored and embraced.

Unique challenges of parenting

Physician parents are in an unique position as they promote and monitor their children's health and development. Their knowledge about health is valuable and helpful, but—as is the case with any parent—their objectivity is limited. It is essential that they ensure their children have a primary care provider who is skilled and comfortable working with the dynamics of physician families. It is also essential that physicians avoid boundary crossings or violations with their children; only in emergencies should they assume a direct clinical role; otherwise, they should join in a collaborative relationship with their child's physician and their child.

Physician parents report that long work hours reduce the quality time they can spend with their children. Where possible, parents should protect structured time to engage with their children, be consistently involved with their children's community, and ensure that a culture of open and welcome communication is fostered. Children will not accept medicine as an excuse for parental distance or under-involvement, nor should they. Besides, spending time with children is a healthy way to remove oneself from the stresses of medical training, return to a world of imagination, creativity and play, and explore the joys of love.

Increasingly, physicians are coupling with other physicians. This creates a remarkably busy family environment that requires careful planning, open communication, flexibility and creativity to manage well. Busy physician parents need to pay particularly good attention to their partner's emotional and physical needs in order to bring richness and closeness to the relationship. Physician parents should be open to seeking counselling should significant relationship difficulties arise: early intervention is associated with high rates of success.

Finally, physicians are high achievers who rarely taste failure. Inadvertently, this can lead to physician parents having unrealistic expectations of their children. Physician parents are well served by engaging in community activities with a diversity of families, monitoring their levels of expectation and approval, and simply enjoying normal development.

How residency programs can help

University programs are encouraged to openly and warmly recognize the universal and unique circumstances and needs of resident physician parents. This may include welcoming family members to program orientation sessions and retreats (with complementary on-site child care available), identification of a staff member well versed in community resources for families (e.g., primary care providers, school advisors, marital/family therapists, recreational centres, babysitters), linkages to nearby daycare and after-hours care facilities, and equitable procedures to address parental leave requests. Family-friendly programs often have an edge in recruiting and retaining excellent residents who, in turn, contribute to the goals of the department in a spirit of collegiality, community and respect.

Case resolution

The resident books a meeting with the program director and formally requested the maximum parental leave open to them. The program director expressed his happiness for the resident and family while indicating that he will respect this request. However, there was one month in particular that posed a challenge in terms of call and clinical coverage, and it was agreed that the resident would work part-time for that one month to facilitate overall leave. This was readily managed with the resident's partner, and everyone was satisfied. Looking back, the resident considers this year of leave one of their best life experiences.

Key references

Dickstein LJ, ed. 1998. *Health Awareness Workshop Reference Manual*. Louisville: Practive Press.

Puddester D. 2004. Staying human in the medical family: the unique role of doctor-parents. *Medical Journal of Australia*. 181 (7): 395–8.

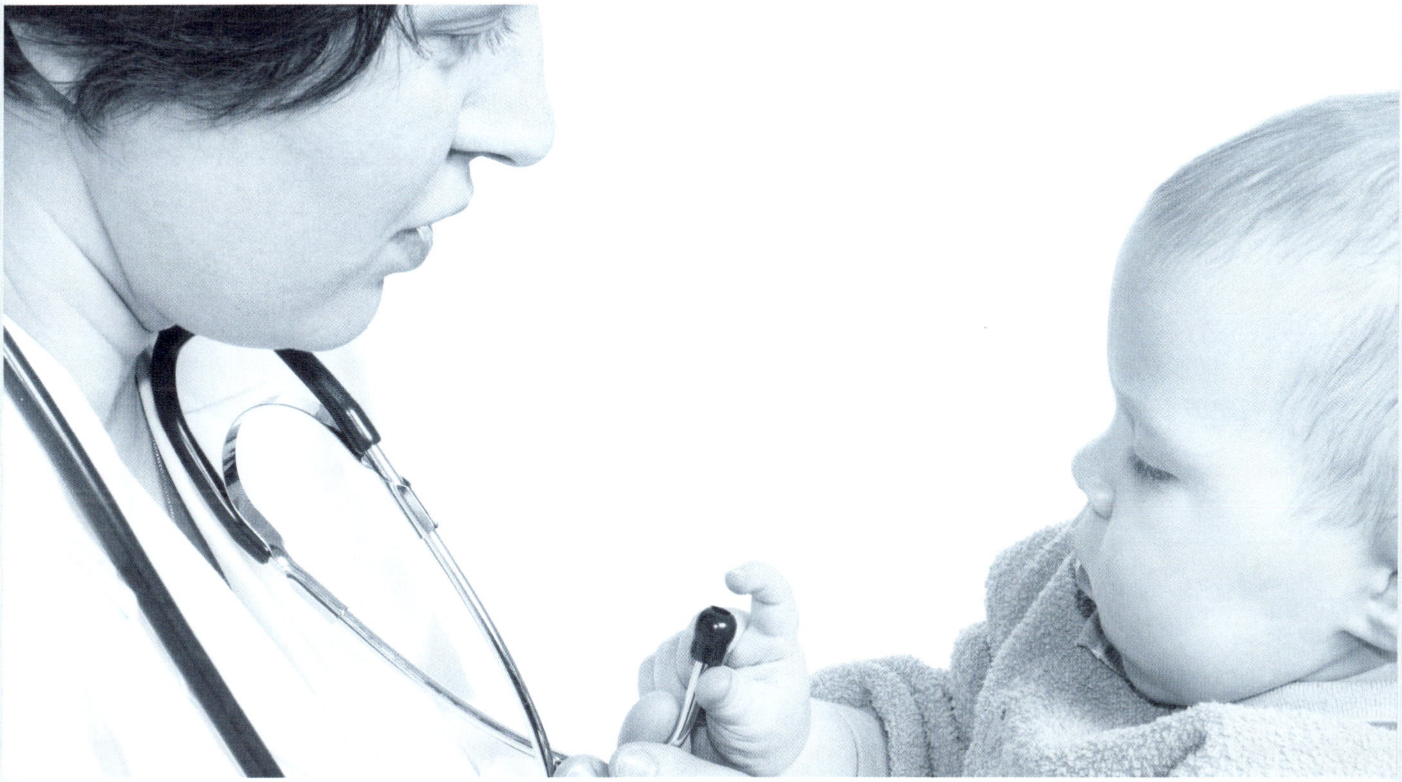

Introduction: Tools for self-care

Leslie Flynn, MD MMus CCFP FRCPC

Most people who choose a career in medicine share hallmark characteristics that have helped them to become high achievers. As a rule, they are energetic, hard-working, enthusiastic, intelligent and self-disciplined. They have learned to delay gratification in the pursuit of their aspirations. They are idealistic, and most come to medicine because they are inspired to contribute to the health and well-being of others.

However, the profession of medicine is demanding, and it is difficult to put limits around its practice. Challenges arise from constant exposure to suffering, heavy workloads, long hours, time pressures, physical and mental demands, and a lack of adequate resources. The stressful nature of the work and of the work environment can take its toll. Physicians are acutely aware of the distress of others but are often less attentive to the stress and fatigue that they experience themselves. Intensive caring for others often leads to neglect of oneself.

We know that physicians, as a group, are well informed with respect to behaviours that contribute to good health. We also know that when physicians are overwhelmed by the demands of their profession, they are vulnerable to neglecting those very behaviours in their own lives. This self-neglect compromises not only the physician's health, but his or her ability to continue to provide care for others.

When self-care is neglected

When a physician becomes immersed in his or her work to the exclusion of self-care, a cascade of stress-induced symptoms generally follows. A feeling of being chronically overwhelmed leads to frustration and irritability. The physician may become prone to emotional outbursts, or may be tearful at work in the face of difficult clinical situations. He or she may take less pleasure in activities that were once much enjoyed. In the meantime, a denial of the significance of these symptoms and the vulnerability they reveal can lead the physician to take on still more work.

Physical symptoms can include intermittent headache, gastrointestinal complaints, and poor sleep, often with a tendency to wake between 2:00 and 4:00 a.m. These symptoms can be accompanied by a change in appetite and a slide into poor eating habits, for example by relying on fast-food outlets rather than taking the time to prepare healthy meals. Energy flags, and a feeling of exhaustion becomes persistent.

When one is feeling emotionally stretched and physically depleted, the thought of exercising is unappealing. Thus physical activity become a low priority, and a lack of healthy exercise erodes one's energy level and sense of well-being even more.

Emotional and physical fatigue lead to behavioural changes. Decreased interest in activities that were once enjoyed during free time leads to social withdrawal and personal isolation. Relationships with family and friends are compromised, and professional interpersonal relationships can be disrupted. Poor coping strategies that are adopted might include the increased intake of caffeine and alcohol, or the use of illicit drugs.

Faced with some or all of these effects, one might experience at the same time a reduced sense of accomplishment and low morale. It is easy to lose sight of one's accomplishments when one is submerged in work. One feels disillusioned and a sense of malaise—if not clear-cut illness. This is the sign of significant stress.

Given that the demands of the profession are ever present, what is the solution? Perhaps it is not as difficult as one might imagine. It requires, first and foremost, awareness of the risks that will be present and deliberate attention to measures of self-care. Physicians' self-care presents a perfect opportunity to practise preventative care.

Solutions: Think "self-care"

In *The 7 Habits of Highly Effective People*, Steven R. Covey makes a compelling case for what he describes as the "Principles of Balanced Self-Renewal," which he describes as "preserving and enhancing the greatest asset you have–you." He identifies four domains that require attention in self-care: physical, emotional, spiritual and mental. Effective self-care requires consideration of these four domains, and taking control of the things that can be controlled.

In caring for one's physical self, planning for healthy eating is a good place to start. We can decide what to eat and when to eat. Taking the time to purchase healthy food and preparing meals that are nutritious will lead to an improved sense of energy and well-being. Planning the use of time away from the workplace, so that exercise is a regular part of one's routine, is also crucial.

There is ample evidence that physical exercise is necessary for both physical and emotional health. Regular exercise is therefore one of the best self-care tools for reducing stress. Choose something that you enjoy. Find someone to join you in the activity and make a commitment to participate regularly. Healthy eating and regular exercise, and minimizing the use of caffeine and alcohol, increases energy, improves outlook and promotes adequate, restorative sleep. Although these strategies for self-care are simple and lie within our control, they are frequently forgotten when we are busy.

Approaching self-care from an emotional perspective begins with recognizing that an exaggerated need for self-sufficiency can lead to loneliness and isolation. Emotional well-being requires that we give ourselves permission to make our own selves a priority. Tending to interpersonal relationships enhances our outlook on life. Protect time in your week to be with others. Value the mutual support that arises from collegial relationships. Spend time with family and friends, sharing laughter and play. Learn strategies such as relaxation techniques to help build the emotional resilience that will be needed in times of stress.

Attending to one's spirituality can take a different form for each person. The essence of this is to learn to listen to one's authentic self. What are your values? What truly inspires and motivates you? To what are you willing to commit your life? Answers to these questions guide each of us in our pursuit of a meaningful life. Adopting a sense of one's spiritual being demands thoughtful attention.

Tools for cognitive well-being include strategies that use the intellect to stimulate thinking, and hence one's outlook, in positive ways. Reading for pleasure provides an escape from the daily grind. Journal writing is a great stress reducer. Writing down your feelings can help you to slow down and reflect on your life and practice. Journal writing can be done on a daily or weekly basis. Learning to set limits on your time and to use time wisely is a cognitive strategy to deliberately attend to self-care. Planning time and space to recharge is an exercise worthy of dedicated attention. Daily, weekly and annual "time outs" are in order.

Summary

The tools for self-care are evident to most physicians: their expertise concerns, after all, what is required to lead a healthy life. However, although they apply this knowledge on a daily basis to guide and educate their patients, under the pressure of their own multiple obligations physicians often find that self-care drops to the bottom of their priority list. Recognizing that self-care, and employing the tools necessary to attend to one's own needs, is not only wise: it is essential to sustain an effective professional life.

Key references

Covey SR. 1989. *The 7 Habits of Highly Effective People*. New York: Simon & Schuster.

Sotile WM and MO Sotile. 2002. *The Resilient Physician: Effective Emotional Management for Doctors and Their Medical Organizations*. Chicago: American Medical Association.

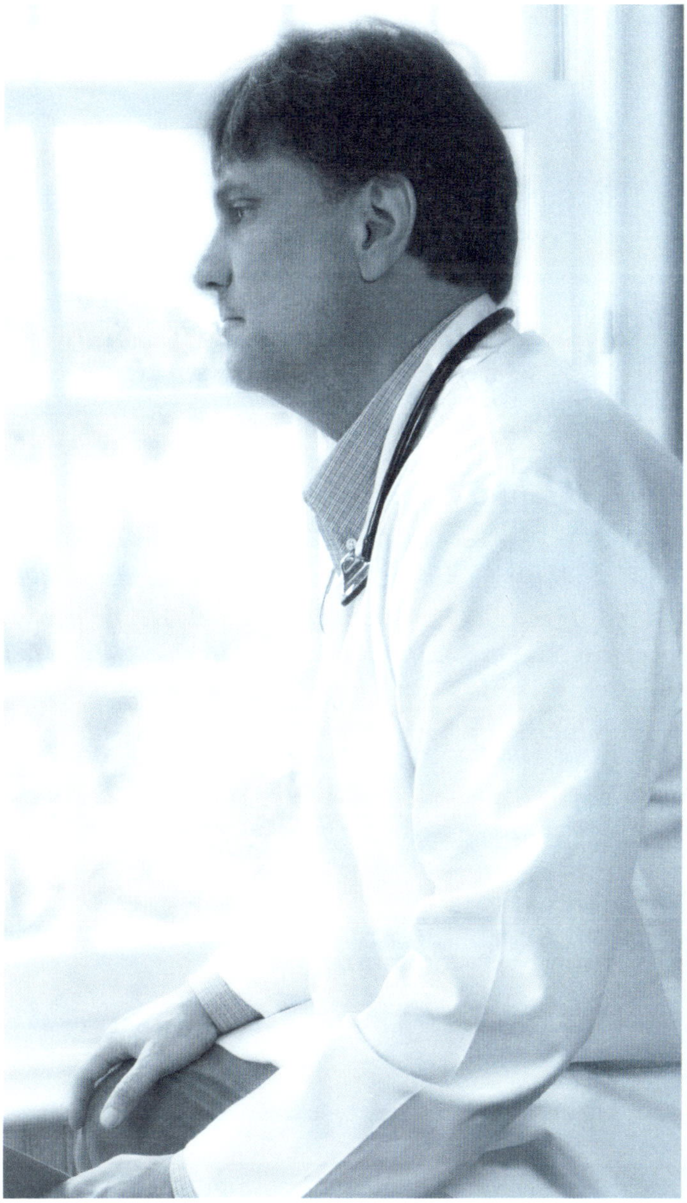

A. Mindfulness and stress management

John Smythe, MD BA FRCPC

Objectives

This chapter will

- describe the basic concept of mindfulness,
- outline a few techniques to cultivate mindfulness, and
- consider ways to incorporate these techniques into daily routines.

> **Case**
>
> A third-year resident has suffered from anxiety throughout their medical training. In the past year, fear of being less competent than their peers has made the anxiety particularly acute. The resident falls into a pattern of daily bingeing and purging as a way to cope with stress. The resident hides this behaviour from others, as they consider the anxiety and bulimia a further sign of inadequacy. However, the resident does enter an introductory six-week mindfulness program offered by the medical school.

Introduction

The road to independent medical practice is long, demanding and fraught with stress. How residents manage their stress largely determines how much they enjoy this period of their lives. Many manage the inevitable stress of their residency years by focusing on the "light at the end of the tunnel," thus continuing a pattern learned even before acceptance into medical school: "If I can only get in, then everything will work out." For the sake of this goal, personal time, relationships, sleep and other needs are deferred. And, of course, after acceptance the workload increases: "Oh well, it will be different in residency; I'll be making money and can finally focus on my real vocation." But residency brings with it a whole new set of demands and stressors, and again one persuades oneself that "real life" can begin "later."

Postponing certain choices today for the promises of tomorrow often makes sense. If we don't crack the books until the week before our fellowship exams, well, we know how that will turn out. But, while planning for the future is helpful, living for it is unhealthy. What's the difference? Planning for the future means orienting our actions so that they contribute to a desired outcome. Living for the future means ignoring how we feel now with the hope that things will be better once we get "there." This amounts to self-neglect.

Managing stress with mindfulness

This habit of living for tomorrow is a flawed coping strategy: it is based on the false premise that tomorrow is more real than today. Today or, more precisely, this moment, is the only moment we exist in. Clearly, the content of this moment is always shifting and new; however, whatever happens, we experience it now. Therefore managing our stress is something we do now or not at all. What is central to stress management is the attention we give ourselves in the present moment.

Paying attention to what we are doing, while we are doing it, is called mindfulness. It is useful to consider how mindful we usually are. Do we pay attention to each bite of our breakfast, or do we hurry it down with gulps of coffee while scanning our emails, half-listening to the radio in the background? Do we carefully listen to our patient's complaints, or are we mostly focused on getting through the patient list in time for handover? For most of us mindlessness is the norm. But mindfulness is not something foreign; it's a capacity we often use. It is both the ability to focus on this text as we read it, and the aspect of mind that notices when our attention has drifted away. Mindfulness is not thinking: it's more like the awareness in which our thoughts and perceptions arise. Deepening our mindfulness through practise is a way of inoculating ourselves against stress.

The relaxation response

We can't avoid stress: stress is triggered by change, and life is change. Nothing is ever settled. When residents eventually finish their training, new challenges will come. But just as we can prepare for an exam by studying, we can prepare for the inevitable presence of stress by practising being present. Stress triggers a predictable cascade of physiological reactions called the stress response. This includes augmented sympathetic output and increases in muscle tension, pulse rate, blood pressure and stress hormone levels. A considerable body of research demonstrates that mindfulness techniques produces a relaxation response that has the opposite effect of the stress response, quieting the autonomic nervous system and lowering the physiological impact of stress. The depth of this physiological quieting significantly exceeds that which occurs in any other state, including sleep.

> **Reflection: Practising mindfulness in daily life**
>
> - Allow yourself a few mindful breaths in the morning before you get out of bed.
> - Try preparing and eating your breakfast quietly, without distraction, once a week.
> - Notice your environment.
> - Drive the speed limit and stop on orange lights.
> - A few times during the day, stop, take a few breaths, and re-center yourself.
> - Let the world wake you up: when you notice a phone ring, a door slam, and so on, take a moment to sense where you are and how you feel.
> - Sign up for a class on meditation, yoga, tai chi, etc.

Exercising mindfulness

Mindfulness can be practised in two ways: informally, through mindful attention during daily activities, and formally, as through structured meditation exercises. Cultivating mindfulness through regular formal practise extends the habit of being present into our daily activities. Try this for the next few breaths. Place one hand on your solar plexus. Notice your abdomen moving in and out with each breath and stay with that sensation. Before long your mind will likely drift off into thoughts about this experience, or about something completely unrelated. When you notice that your mind has drifted into thinking, let go of the thoughts and come back to the sense of breathing. Practise this for a few minutes. It's simple and yet difficult to stay present: it takes discipline to train our minds to simply be in the moment when our tendency is to want to control it.

Making friends with fear

Stress arises from our attempt to create certainty in an uncertain world. This anxiety often causes us to avoid our feelings (e.g., procrastinating, "vegging out" in front of the television) or to try to control them (e.g., endlessly making lists, incessantly checking email). Such activities might take the edge off our anxiety momentarily, but when anxiety has the upper hand in our lives the activities that are motivated by anxiety become deeply entrenched habits. To manage stress effectively we must properly confront our fears. Mindfulness is the key to doing so.

In a state of mindfulness we allow ourselves to feel whatever arises within us. Whether we are feeling overwhelmed by anger or lost in boredom we simply allow ourselves to be aware of our experience. By staying with uncomfortable feelings, making room for these natural human experiences, we lessen their control over us. When the code pager goes off, while a flurry of thoughts and feelings may flood through us, our patience and experience allow us to approach these situations with a calm, sensible responsiveness. With mindfulness training, we can learn to stay present with our feelings and let go of the thoughts that normally ensnare us when our fear or impatience erupts.

Case resolution

Working with the mindfulness techniques of meditation, body scanning and yoga, the resident is able after a few weeks to delay, and eventually eliminate, the binging episodes. The resident also begins to question these negative self-judgments and seeks counselling for the eating problems and low self-esteem. The resident discloses these challenges and fears to a close friend and feels less isolated and less anxious about life in general. The resident plans to continue with regular meditation.

Self-acceptance

As we become mindful of uncomfortable feelings and the habitual patterns they trigger, we may become self-critical: "I can't believe I was so sensitive (or so insensitive)." But the point of mindfulness is to accept, not judge, ourselves. Cranky or tired, sexually restless or serene, what matters is that we can deepen our capacity to notice, and to be with, whatever arises. Self-acceptance is the basis of self-esteem. It gives us the confidence to be genuine and to live with authenticity. As we become more familiar with our own nature, more accepting of our quirks and foibles, we also naturally become more accepting of others. In medical practice there is no greater kindness we can offer our patients than our attention and acceptance. Thus, mindfulness practice is a kindness that we offer ourselves, but that benefits others as well.

Key references

Hassed C, de Lisle S, Sullivan G, Pier C. 2008 Enhancing the health of medical students: outcomes of an integrated mindfulness and lifestyle program. *Advances in Health Sciences Education.* In Press.

Kabat-Zinn J. 1994. *Wherever You Go, There You Are: Mindfulness Meditation in Everyday Life.* New York: Hyperion Press.

Wicks RJ. 2007. *The Resilient Clinician.* New York: Oxford University Press.

B. Journal writing

Helga Ehrlich, MD CCFP FCFP

Objectives

This chapter will

- outline the benefits of keeping a journal in guiding self-reflection,
- discuss how keeping a journal can help clarify values and beliefs, and hence our responses to situations, and
- demonstrate how writing can help us slow down, focus, and attend to the emotions we are experiencing.

Case

A second-year resident began their cardiology rotation two weeks ago. The resident has just had a particularly stressful week with more than the usual number of admissions. Early in the second week the resident admitted a 53-year-old architect to the coronary care unit with the diagnosis of a second myocardial infarction. The patient had been well until shortly before his 49th birthday, when he began to experience anginal pain. One month later he suffered his first heart attack. His recovery proceeded without complication, and he returned to work within approximately three months. This second heart attack, four years later, has caused the patient a great deal of anxiety, and he no longer wants to adhere to any treatment regimens.

The resident feels threatened and uncertain about how to proceed, given the patient's apathy. During cardiology rounds with the staff cardiologist, various medical data are reviewed and a vigorous debate ensues among team members regarding the appropriate thrombolytic therapy for the patient. The resident realizes during the course of daily assessments and interactions with the patient that, as a resident, they feel increasingly frustrated and at a loss as to how to reach the patient.

The following week, overtired but determined, the resident finally breaks through. The resident ends up asking the patient what it was like having suffered yet another health setback in the prime of his career and with a relatively young family.

Introduction

Medical practice has always been grounded in life's intersubjective domain. It unfolds in a series of complex clinical encounters involving narratives—stories in which one human being listens and extends help to another. Like narrative, medical practice requires the engagement of one person with another and realizes that authentic engagement is transformative for all participants (Charon 2001).

As a result of research in patient-centred communication and an increased interest in the medical humanities, the art of medicine has become more sophisticated with respect to narrative modes of knowing and the narratives of patients and physicians in particular. Through narrative, practitioners can better understand the experiences of their patients as well as their own journeys as physicians (Charon 2004). One route to that understanding is to chronicle the experiences we share with our patients.

A journal of the grieving process

Dr. Milne was going through a complicated grieving process. She was distressed by the loss of two young patients, from two very different families, who had died during the same week. She began to write intermittently in a journal, describing her thoughts and interpretations of these difficult events. She purposefully wrote without much forethought, letting the words flow, letting her feelings bubble up to the surface.

She described the rooms where Jason and Steven had died and was surprised at how vividly she remembered certain details: Jason's fish tank, the morning light filtering through the curtains onto Steven's tired face, the muted sounds, the encounters with various family members.

She recalled how she had bought a large bouquet of helium balloons on her way home from work the day after Jason died. She was coming home to her two-year-old daughter, and to her son, who was Jason's age. She wanted to deliver to her own children some emblem of joyfulness and hope, and something that pointed toward heaven.

In the weeks that followed, Dr. Milne occasionally reread her journal entries, adding more recollections. This process allowed her to reflect on her responses and to consider her personal reasons for feeling so overwhelmed at the time. She was aware of how much she identified with Jason's family and also how much she would miss seeing Steven and his family. In articulating these thoughts, she learned to be more patient with herself. She also began to speak with a more experienced colleague about how she was handling things. She realized that these memories were important to her, and that the act of writing them down, had given her more insight, more acceptance of her emotions, and a measure of comfort as well.

Discussion

Medicine is a relationship-based profession. Physicians engaged in clinical care are inevitably affected by the complexities of patient care: joy, suffering, courage, loss and love. As reflective practitioners, we learn to identify and interpret our emotional responses to patients and in doing so are able to "make sense of their life journeys and grant what is called for—and called forth"—in facing ill and vulnerable patients (Charon 2006).

On some level, physicians grieve along with their patients; they are "aware of how disease changes everything, what it means, what it claims, how random is its unfairness and how much courage it takes to look it full in the face." (DasGupta 2006). The textbox gives an example of how keeping a journal can assist in this emotional process.

Summary

Writing in a journal can help us to bridge professional and personal gaps. The kinesthetic exercise of writing and also of close reading allows physicians to do what medical sociologist Arthur Frank calls "thinking with stories." In his words, "To think about a story is to reduce it to its content and then analyze that content [...] To think with a story is to experience it affecting one's own life and to find in that effect a certain truth of one's own life."

Journal entries can give shape to clinical experiences so that they can be seen and understood by both the writer and audience. "The previously formless experience thereby becomes like an edifice, around which the writer can walk, seeing it from all directions, understanding aspects that, until form was conferred, were invisible" (Frank 1995). By chronicling our experiences as physicians, we learn the value of telling and retelling, of gaining understanding, and of respecting and learning from the many authentic stories we share.

Case resolution

The patient hesitated but then, with relief, talked about his fear of failure and his fear of dying. He spoke of his anger and resentment of being afflicted with a life-threatening illness so early in his productive years. He did not want people's sympathy, nor did he want to be a burden to anyone. By the time the resident was completing the cardiology rotation and was following the patient in cardiac rehabilitation, the patient was noticeably better in terms of mood and in his acceptance that lifestyle changes would be permanent. He was better able to discuss the actual experience of cardiac illness. The resident learns the therapeutic value of talking with a patient about his illness and, by doing so, helping to order that experience for both patient and physician.

Key references

Charon R. 2001. Narrative medicine. A model for empathy, reflection, profession, and trust. *Journal of the American Medical Association*. 286: 1897–902.

Charon R. 2004. Narrative and medicine. *New England Journal of Medicine*. 350 (9): 862–4.

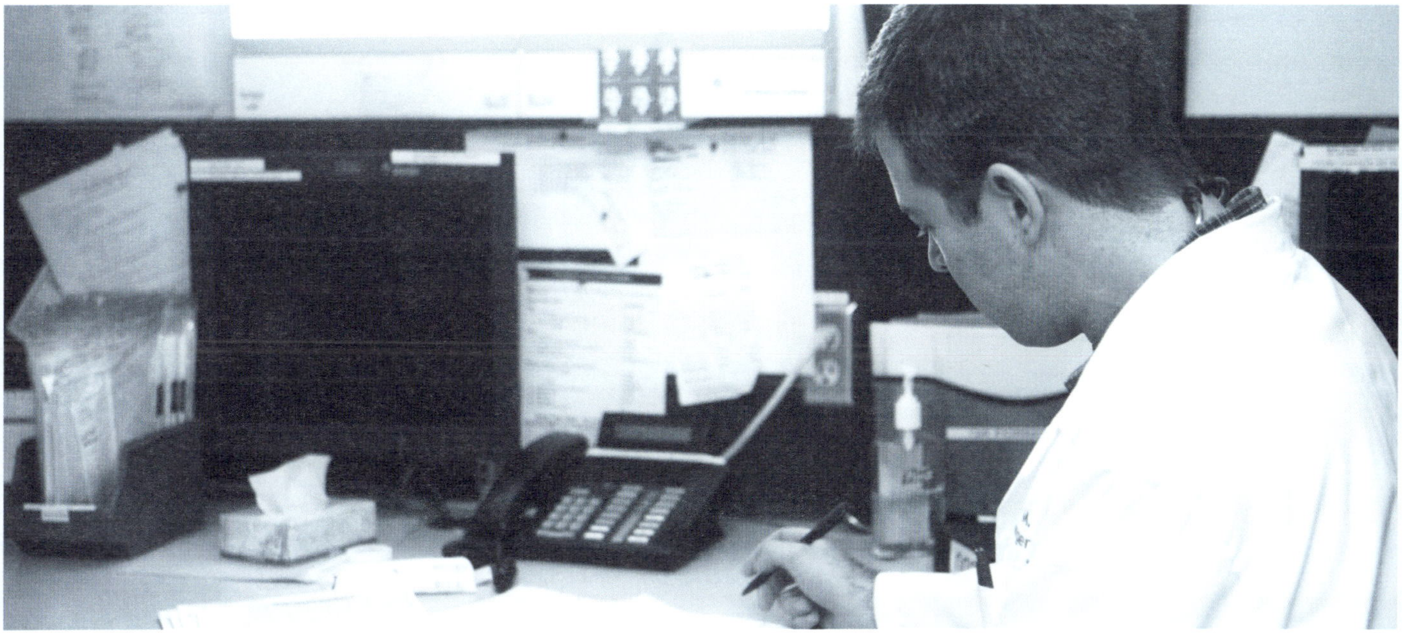

C. Exercise and physical fitness

Andrew Pipe, CM MD LLD(Hon) DSc(Hon)

Objectives

This chapter will

- present evidence of the benefits of regular physical activity,
- describe the importance of integrating regular physical activity into one's lifestyle, and
- discuss the importance of modelling being physically active to colleagues, students and the medical community.

Case

A fourth-year resident recognizes that they are more breathless than before when climbing stairs. Always physically active throughout their teens, as an undergraduate and medical student, the resident realizes that over the four years of the postgraduate program they have become increasingly sedentary. The demands of work and the need to spend time with their partner and young daughter seem to have eliminated the cherished private time when they would jog to and from the hospital as a student and first-year resident.

Introduction

Evidence of the health benefits of physical activity is long-standing, incontrovertible and ever-increasing. Regular participation in physical activity greatly decreases the likelihood of chronic disease and premature mortality. All physicians acknowledge the powerful role that exercise can play in developing and accentuating health in every dimension. Unfortunately, despite this knowledge, physicians appear to be no more active than the population as a whole. And, sadly, although medical students are typically active on a regular basis, it is too often the case that as they embark upon their careers they give less time to personal physical activity.

The challenges of professional and personal life, constraints of time, and the frequently self-imposed pressures of conflicting responsibilities and obligations can significantly reduce the likelihood that regular physical activity will be part of a physician's lifestyle. At the same time, many medical practitioners bring to exercise the same achievement-oriented, goal-driven approach that is in part responsible for their success as students and physicians. However, while an athletic model of physical activity may be motivating and rewarding for some, it is daunting for many. It is reassuring to know that the health benefits of physical activity accrue with as little as thirty minutes of moderate-intensity exercise most days of the week. The evidence also reveals that physicians who are themselves active are much more likely to counsel their patients about the important, health-enhancing properties of an active lifestyle.

Description

Moderate physical activity can result in better general health (health-related fitness); more intense activity will increase athletic capacity (performance-related fitness). Many people do not appreciate that the multiple health benefits of regular physical activity—enhanced cardio-respiratory and musculo-skeletal performance, reduced likelihood of obesity, diabetes, circulatory disorders, depression, anxiety and osteoporosis—are associated with regular, physical activity of moderate intensity. It is not necessary to become an athlete to enjoy the significant rewards of physical activity. The benefits of sustained, moderate-intensity aerobic activity are protean and go well beyond improving cardiovascular health. Regular physical activity can be a time for recreation—in the fullest sense. Thirty minutes spent walking, biking, jogging, swimming or skating can permit an escape from pagers, telephones and the pressures of practice and provide an opportunity for retreat and reflection. Predictably, perhaps, some physicians apply an academic perspective to physical activity and seek to calculate training heart rates and intensity-duration schedules: an approach suited to athletic training, but not necessary to enhance overall health. The so-called "talk test" (exercising at an intensity that permits simple conversation with an exercising partner or friend) is a remarkably accurate indicator of a level of activity that optimizes cardio-respiratory function and other aspects of health.

The challenges are obvious. How does the busy practitioner protect sufficient time for physical exercise? How can one integrate physical activity into one's personal and professional lifestyle? How do we normalize such activity within the professional community? Following the "Four F's" can provide a practical framework for achieving these goals; physical activity should be: *fun*, *feasible*, include *family and friends*, and continue *forever*.

Fun. Physical activity must be enjoyable. Activities that are tedious, uncomfortable or intimidating are not likely to form the basis of a lifetime of healthy physical activity. Find something you enjoy and look forward to the release it offers from the pressures of a busy professional life.

Feasible. Activities that require elaborate equipment, specialized facilities or significant travel are difficult to integrate into daily life. A lunchtime walk, an evening jog, or a regular swim or aerobics session at a nearby "Y" requires little equipment and minimal preparation and can be integrated easily into daily routines. Biking to work and taking the stairs whenever possible will add to the ease with which physical activity can be included in daily schedules.

Family and friends. Physical activity that frequently involves family and friends has a further motivation built in. Encouraging the whole family to engage in regular physical activity can allow you to pass on your exercise "values" to your children, optimizing their growth and development. Skiing, biking, sledding, hiking—he choices are limitless.

Forever. Participation in physical activity is for life. Establishing favourite physical activities early in a career helps to ensure that enjoyable, anticipated and active periods will be integrated into weekly rhythms for the long term. Realistic expectations of exercise intensity will help prevent injury and increase the likelihood of enjoyable physical recreation over a lifetime.

Summary

Regular physical activity is life-enhancing. In addition to the benefits to physical health, physical activity allows private, personal time for reflection and recreation. It is important for physicians to integrate physical activity into their personal lifestyles in ways that are both practical and, most importantly, pleasurable.

Key references

Frank E, Breyan J, Elon L. 2000. Physician disclosure of healthy personal behaviors improves credibility and ability to motivate. *Archives of Family Medicine.* 9: 287–90.

Gaertner PH, Firor WB, Edouard L. 1991. Physical inactivity among physicians. *Canadian Medical Association Journal.* 144: 1253–6.

Case resolution

Deciding to make one's personal health a priority is an important step in making time for physical activity. There will always be rounds to attend and journals to read, and demands on a young resident's time are seemingly inexhaustible. By thoughtfully scheduling clinical and study time, recognizing the realities of an on-call schedule, and discussing these issues with resident colleagues, this resident is able to incorporate regular physical activity into their lifestyle. The resident no longer takes elevators unless absolutely necessary (there's a "Stairway to Health" program in the hospital), the resident bikes to work two days a week, attends a weekly yoga class at the local "Y", and a Saturday morning swim or walk with family is now a regular part of weekends when the resident is not on call. As chief resident, they also encourage younger colleagues to look after themselves in a similar manner. Family vacations are now chosen with physical activities in mind: camping and canoeing in the summer.

By demonstrating to friends and colleagues that physical activity is important to one's well-being, the resident ensures understanding and support as they optimize time for personal health. (The department chief has also taken up biking to work and is a new convert to physician health! His welcoming address to new residents now includes supportive advice on the importance of personal health and physical activity). Both the resident and fellow residents understand that in certain circumstances it may be necessary to depart from this schedule. The resident's bicycle helmet serves as a reminder to colleagues, hospital and attending staff that personal health and physical activity are important, central components of a contemporary practitioner's lifestyle.

The resident's example and leadership result in the hospital providing bike racks and shower facilities for staff. Next month, at the annual refresher course, the resident has been asked to lead a morning session of the CMA's "Walk the Doc" program for all participants.

D. Spirituality

John Smythe, MD BA FRCPC

Objectives

This chapter will

- introduce a model of considering the role of spirituality in the process of care,
- encourage consideration of spirituality in the promotion of physician health and well-being, and
- offer tools and methods to reflect on one's spiritual resiliance.

> **Case**
> A first-year resident is feeling disillusioned with medicine. The resident entered medicine because their father died of lung cancer when the resident was in high school. Now feeling frustrated by the inevitable deaths of too many of their patients the resident is thinking of taking a year off to reconsider their options.

Introduction

At heart, spiritual practice is about noticing life as we live it. The wisdom and compassion that this engenders does not make us more expert; it makes us more human. Science teaches us how to *do;* spirituality, how to *be.* As physicians, we can benefit from practising both.

Courses on spirituality have begun to appear in medical school curricula. However, considerable controversy remains as to the relevance of spirituality in medicine. Spirituality is primarily an inner, subjective matter, whereas Western medicine is based on objective, empirical science. Whether or not spiritual matters belong in our medical curricula, surveys suggest that most medical practitioners do consider spiritual questions and values personally relevant. For example, compassion, a principle central to all spiritual traditions, is embedded in the practise of good medical care. Interestingly, there is now some research evidence that the empathy and compassion typical of newly enrolled medical students become less apparent by the end of fourth-year clerkship (Newton et al 2008). Perhaps this is because the scientific and pragmatic knowledge acquired during training, together with the stresses of medical training, result in an "objectification" of patients which may make us less sensitive and available to people in their suffering. That is to say, caring as empathetic concern is gradually replaced by caring as a means to an end: freedom from disease. Yet these two aspects of caring, the spiritual and the material, are not mutually exclusive.

From the spiritual perspective, one could say that caring is not so much a means to an end as an end in itself. Spirituality is fundamentally about a sense of connection to someone or something other than oneself. In medicine, when caring for others, we have the opportunity to deepen this sense of connection by openly and honestly relating to our patients. Yet this is challenging and potentially exhausting work. And it is a practice that requires ongoing self-reflection and attention.

Compassion fatigue

Sadly, one sometimes hears of dedicated, compassionate physicians, unfailing in their commitment to patients and the profession, who take their own life. How does this happen? In medicine we have an Achilles heel. We tend to forget to care for ourselves when we are single-mindedly committed to the ideal of caring for others. Compassion that does not include oneself is incomplete. And it often leads to burnout.

Burnout is distressingly common in medicine, as in other occupations where time is spent supporting others. Burnout sufferers describe feelings of isolation, depersonalization and emotional exhaustion—or "compassion fatigue"—associated with a sense of reduced personal accomplishment. They have what might be regarded as a spiritual illness: if engagement with one's life is a sign of spiritual health, burnout is the opposite. Physicians who were once wholeheartedly committed to medicine begin to avoid work, become less interested in their patients, and doubt their career choice.

Not surprisingly, burnout can lead to depression, addiction and suicide. How does caring for others come to this? The altruistic ideals, long hours, tensions between personal and work obligations, and historical insensitivity of the medical profession to the health of its members all contribute to the psychological and emotional vulnerability of physicians. This vulnerability is intensified in residency by the lack of a sense of personal control inherent in junior positions. Given that burnout is an occupational risk for physicians, how can they lessen it? One important way is to develop spiritual resilience.

Spiritual resilience and self-awareness

Immunizing ourselves against the inevitable stresses of our profession requires us to regularly nourish the spirit. One essential means of doing this is to deepen self-awareness by consciously paying attention to our own selves. There is much talk these days about the importance of balance. Diet, exercise, relationships, study, play, work—these all need to be integrated into a balanced whole. But who decides on the relative weight we place on each aspect of this whole, and how do we know when we are out of balance? We do, through self-reflection.

Balance doesn't derive from a checklist, nor can it be conferred by an external authority. It comes from connecting with ourselves and nurturing a sense of groundedness. Being consciously present and patiently attending to our own state of mind and body helps us to recentre ourselves when we feel off-balance. Perhaps we are feeling completely frustrated with the cardiac patient we've been called to see for the fourth time today. Perhaps we'd rather ignore the pager altogether, or unload on the clerk who keeps paging us. Instead, just stopping for a few moments and letting ourselves honestly feel our frustration and fatigue may be what we really need.

When we notice difficult feelings and still accept ourselves, without self-criticism or denial, we are developing compassion for ourselves. We all experience aspects of ourselves that we'd prefer to root out or ignore. But openness and self-acceptance are the basis of compassion. As we connect honestly and openly with ourselves it becomes easier to be available in this way for others. Mindfully listening to a patient's anxieties is natural for those who've made room in their hearts for their own fears.

Reflection: Suggestions for spiritual well-being

- **Connect with your purpose.** What matters to you? What touches your heart? Purpose is an energizing force. It inspires and invigorates.
- **Connect with the moment.** When you are washing your hands between patients, notice the specific way you move them, the sensation of the water, its temperature, and the slipperiness of soap. Sense your feet on the ground, and the environment around you.
- **Connect with yourself.** It is easy to lose your centre when attending to other people and concerns all day. Taking time every day to quietly reflect, write, or just be present, can bring you back to yourself.
- **Practice gratitude.** Recall something that you are grateful for at the end of each day.
- **Keep your sense of humour.** A light touch can provide perspective.

Spiritual opportunities

People have a natural resistance to being open: we fear that it will make us vulnerable. It takes courage to be open and to care: it is challenging and sometimes painful work. We generally prefer the presumed security of certainty, of knowing how things should be rather than experiencing how things actually are. So, rather than being open to ourselves and our life, we may constantly try to manage everything. But when life brings something clearly unmanageable to our doorstep, what then? We fail to get into the program we want; someone we love leaves us or is diagnosed with a terminal illness; our patient unexpectedly dies. When life overwhelms our efforts to control it, we have a spiritual opportunity.

From a spiritual perspective, openness to life in all of its expressions, painful or otherwise, is the path. Beyond our agendas of controlling every outcome, or curing every disease, lie many spiritual opportunities: to be touched by the unspeakable rawness of a mother's grief over her lost child; to be humbled by the equanimity of our dying cancer patient. We may prefer to avoid or ignore such experiences when they arise and run off to write our notes in the chart. Yet, medicine is a challenging profession in large part because it directly exposes us to the entire human condition. It doesn't allow us to hide from suffering or from joy. And it is precisely because of this that physicians often find spiritual practices of deep benefit.

Finding and using practices that connect us with our experiences, from writing in a journal to contemplation to meditation, can help keep us grounded. By coming back to our own sense of presence, we are then more able to be present to others. Our willingness to connect with ourselves thus becomes a stepping-stone to a deeper connection with our patients and our world.

Case resolution

The resident mentions these feelings to a hospital chaplain, with whom a dialogue on death and dying begins. The resident realizes that they hadn't really dealt with their father's death and so joins a bereavement group. This allows the resident to get in touch with their anger and sorrow. The resident begins to feel less isolated and finds it easier to relate to what patients and their families are experiencing. The resident now makes a conscious effort to notice things that they are grateful for. The resident thinks they will remain in medicine.

Key references

Curlin FA, Lantos JD, Roach CJ, Sellergren SA, Chin MH. 2005. Religious characteristics of U.S. physicians: A national survey. *Journal of General Internal Medicine.* 20: 629–34.

Kearney MK, Weininger RB, Vachon MLS, Harrison RL, Mount BM. 2009. Self-care of physicians caring for patients at the end of life: "Being connected ... a key to my survival." *Journal of the American Medical Association.* 301: 1155–64.

Larimore WL, Duininck MW, Morsch GB. 2007. Spiritual needs of physicians during and following a catastrophe. *Southern Medical Journal.* 100 (9): 940–1.

Newton B, Barber L, Clardy J, Cleveland E, O'Sullivan P. 2008. Is there hardening of the heart during medical school? *Academic Medicine.* March; 83(3): 244-9.

E. Finding a family physician

Lee Donohue, MD MHSc

Objectives

This chapter will

- explore strategies and resources for obtaining a personal family physician, and
- discuss some of the barriers that limit physician consultations with a family physician.

> **Case**
>
> A third-year resident has used the birth control pill previously and wants to begin again. She chooses a package from the samples that are available at the community office where she works.
>
> The resident is your colleague and does not have a personal family physician. Does she need one? Do you know how to help her to find one? Review the regulations or recommendations of your licensing college that relate to this case.
>
> Now pretend that you are the resident's personal family physician. Do you agree or disagree with her decision. If so, why?

Introduction

What factors influence physicians to consult another physician on matters concerning their own health? Are these factors different from those that prompt other patients to see a doctor?

In general, despite heavy workloads and responsibilities, physicians are as healthy as the general population. Like other patients, physician patients most often choose self-care for common illnesses and concerns. Occasionally, such as in an emergency or when a surgical or technical procedure is required, there is no choice but to consult another physician. In other situations a consultation may occur because the physician patient or physician parent acknowledges that he or she has insufficient objectivity to make an informed choice. At other times the decision to consult will fall into a "gray zone," much like the physician in the case experienced, where the self-care decision may seem straightforward for the physician patient, except for the fact that, for any other patient a visit to a physician to obtain a consultation, prescription or a signed requisition would be required.

Physicians needing physicians

Research is lacking on the decision-making processes that doctors use to determine when and with whom they should consult about personal or family health issues. In Canada, access to a family physician is a problem for all patients, including physician patients.

Some common questions for physician patients include:

- From whom should I obtain medical care? Do I need a specialist in family medicine or is it better for me to see a surgeon or internist directly?
- How can I find a family physician?

We do not have objective measures of what doctors need from their personal physicians, nor do we know whether their needs differ from those of other patients. However, there is good evidence that access to a family physician helps to maximize health. Family medicine is comprehensive, longitudinal, patient- and family-centred care. A family physician considers the whole picture of the health needs of the patient and not just the presenting symptom or concern.

A family physician functions as a personal health care consultant for you and your family. A family physician can diagnose and treat the entire range of your health problems, or refer you appropriately to a consultant. Your family physician keeps a record of your personal and family health issues and provides health education, prevention and screening advice. A family physician is an expert in coordination of care to ensure that all your health needs are considered. Most importantly, your personal family physician assists you with decisions about your health and health care services.

How can you find a family physician?

- Ask your friends, colleagues, your chief of staff, or your local medical society for the names of physicians who are accepting new patients.
- See the same family doctor that your spouse and children see.
- Look out of town: some physicians prefer to have a non-local family physician.
- If you are moving to a new region, ask your previous family physician to recommend a family physician in that area.
- Call your provincial physician health program for suggestions. Contact information is available at: www.cma.ca/physicianhealth
- Find out if your employer, health region or medical society has a program that will help you find a family physician. If not, advocate for such a service.

Unlike other patients, physicians can access the health care system and self-diagnose, self-refer and self-prescribe; traditionally, however, they have been implored not to do so, but to behave like "normal" patients and seek treatment recommendations from others rather than directing their own care. Nowadays, as a result of improved access to medical information, a growing emphasis on collaborative care, and fiscal realities, the paradigm of care is shifting to encourage greater patient autonomy, informed decision-making, increased self-care and a more active role for patients in treatment decisions. These four characteristics have always been commonplace in the care of physician patients. However, the shift from paternalistic care toward shared decision-making, which includes consideration of research evidence, risks and benefits, and patient needs and values, nonetheless applies to the treatment of physicians.

Building a good family physician relationship

Robert Lamberts, a physician based in Augusta, Georgia, has written a list of rules to assist him to get along with his patients and for his patients to get along with him. Consider these as you interact with your family physician, and as you care for patients, including your physician colleagues.

Rules for patients to get along with their doctor:

- **Rule 1:** Your doctor can't do it alone.
- **Rule 2:** Be honest.
- **Rule 3:** Your doctor can't play favourites.
- **Rule 4:** Don't mess with the staff.
- **Rule 5:** If you don't trust, leave. Trusting a doctor does not mean you should not ask questions. Questioning is often the only way to build trust.

distractible.org/2008/08/11/getting-along-part-2-patient-rules/

Rules for doctors to get along with their patients:

- **Rule 1:** They don't want to be at your office. Show compassion.
- **Rule 2:** They have a reason to be at your office. Try to identify the real reason (or the real fear) that brings them into your office.
- **Rule 3:** They feel what they feel. You have to trust your patient.
- **Rule 4:** They don't want to look stupid.
- **Rule 5:** They want to know what is going to be done and when.
- **Rule 6:** The visit is about them.

distractible.org/2008/08/06/getting-along-part-1-doctor-rules/

In a shared-decision-making model of care, both the patient and physician work together to decide about screening, prevention, diagnosis and treatment. It is patient-centred, involving the patient in whatever decisions are made. This does not mean that the patient must always agree with the physician's recommendation, or that the physician must agree with the patient's preferences. Rather, the treating physician and the physician patient find concordance on an approach to care in illness and in health. In this partnership, as the physician patient you must decide how much participation to seek from the other doctor in the room, your personal physician. Your personal physician must do the same and negotiate how much participation from you, the patient, will assist with quality decision-making and care.

Physicians must seek out best care and be mindful of the benefits and hazards that their knowledge and training bring to their health care decisions. As physician patients we cannot help but approach our personal medical issues with an expert perspective. However, physician expertise does not necessarily assist with decision-making; indeed, clouded by subjective concerns, it can sometimes impair decision-making about personal health issues.

In family medicine, much of our ability to diagnose and advise is based on a trusting relationship with our patients that develops over time as, together, we solve problems. As physician patients all of us need to find opportunities to build that trusting relationship with a family physician. Through these opportunities your personal physician learns how to do a better job in caring for you. As in all relationships, there must be support and resolve to permit the relationship to grow.

As one commentator has written, for there to be a justified trust between patient and doctor, "the consultation must be grounded not on knowledge alone, but also on benevolence between doctor and patient, and on respect by each for the autonomy of the other [...] Justified trust comes from the build up of experience in the responsible and sensitive care of numbers of actual patients: this can be colloquialised as 'part of the job'; but it is also an essential element of professional development" (Black 2000). It is through these trusting relationships that physicians will obtain quality health care for themselves and their families.

Case resolution

The resident used the services available through her local physician health program to find a family physician. At her first visit the resident obtained a prescription for her birth control pills and a lab requisition to screen for sexually transmitted infections, and scheduled a follow-up visit.

Key references

Canadian Physician Health Network. Last retrieved June 25, 2009, from CMA's website: www.cma.ca/index.cfm/ci_id/25567/la_id/1.htm.

Jadad AR, Rizo CA, Enkin MW. 2003. I am a good patient, believe it or not. *BMJ*. 326: 1293–4.

Lussier MT and C Richard. 2008. Because one shoe doesn't fit all: a repertoire of doctor–patient relationships. *Canadian Family Physician*. 54 (8): 1089–92.

F. Nutrition

Jane Lemaire, MD FRCPC; Jean E. Wallace, PhD; Kelly Dinsmore, MSc; and Delia Roberts, PhD.

Objectives

This chapter will

- describe some of the barriers to adequate nutrition in the workplace,
- discuss how inadequate nutrition can affect physicians personally and professionally, and
- suggest ways in which individual physicians can influence workplace wellness.

> **Case**
>
> Over the last two years, a second-year resident has found it increasingly difficult to maintain a nutrition and exercise program. In particular the usual attention to healthy nutrition has been gradually eroded by long sessions in the operating room and lengthy work days. The resident regards the nutrition choices at the hospital as unacceptable and finds they are missing meals, losing weight and generally feeling awful on most days.

Introduction

Although physicians generally have healthy eating habits, they often report that they are unable to eat properly or at all during regular work days and, in particular, during extended on-call hours. When considering physicians' nutrition in the workplace, the solution should be simple—just make time to eat sensibly. However, the issue is not so straightforward, and even though physicians would like to stop and eat or drink, it is often not possible to do so. Many factors can affect physicians' nutrition in the workplace, including the length of routine work days, the frequency of extended or on-call work hours, the urgent nature of practice, the public's expectations of physician performance, and the influence of health care organizations' nutrition resources and policies (e.g., lack of access to nutritional food after hours). Other contributing factors can include personal characteristics such as perfectionist or workaholic traits, and the pressure of stringent professional norms and expectations.

Nutrition in the health care workplace

To improve nutrition in the workplace, physicians and health care organizations must enhance their awareness and understanding of the impact of inadequate nutrition and the barriers to good nutrition. Without this knowledge, there will be little impetus from either group to improve the status quo.

How common are problems with inadequate nutrition? Very. For example, one study provided a description of some of the physical stresses experienced by critical care fellows in training, including evidence of inadequate nutrition: ketonuria, an indicator of poor nutrition, was found in 21 per cent of study participants (Parshuram 2004). Another study demonstrated that only 14 per cent of the participants consumed the recommended six to eight glasses of water per day, and the majority (60 per cent) snacked less than once a day (Winston 2008). A qualitative study in which physicians were interviewed about their workplace nutrition habits reported that 19 of the 20 participants expressed that they sometimes have difficulty eating and drinking during work hours (Lemaire et al 2008). In view of the evolving body of literature supporting a link between physician wellness and quality of patient care, appropriate nutrition during work hours should be recognized as a valid wellness factor.

What is the impact of inadequate nutrition on physicians? Poor nutrition for physicians during the work day has significant consequences, both for the individual physician and for the workplace. Physicians have previously described how their inability to eat and drink properly during work hours is directly related to emotional symptoms such as irritability and frustration, physical symptoms such as being tired, hungry and nauseated, and cognitive symptoms such as the inability

> **Suggestions for improving nutrition in the workplace**
>
> For physicians:
>
> - Eat breakfast.
> - Carry healthy and convenient snacks with you.
> - Schedule nutrition breaks as a priority within your work day (e.g., mid-morning, lunch, mid-afternoon, evening).
> - Plan for a balanced nutritional intake (should include carbohydrates, protein and healthy fats).
> - Learn to recognize the emotional and physical symptoms that declare it's time to eat and drink (irritability, fatigue and hunger pangs).
> - Model and reward healthy nutritional behaviours for your colleagues and trainees, and educate others on the benefits of nutrition breaks for improving performance.
>
> For health care organizations:
>
> - Improve the quality and variety of foods available in the workplace.
> - Improve access to nutritious food (e.g., in the doctors' lounge, near work units, on mobile carts).
> - Provide designated areas where physicians can eat, drink and store food from home.
> - Promote and support a healthy workplace, recognizing that physician wellness is linked to quality of patient care.

to focus, concentrate or think clearly, with resultant poor decision-making and performance (Lemaire et al 2008). They also felt that inadequate nutrition had a negative impact on both their ability to complete their work and on their interactions with patients, colleagues and other health care professionals. In addition, objective testing has shown that physicians who consumed adequate nutrition during a work day had better cognitive function than those who neglected their nutritional needs.

What are the barriers to promoting healthy nutrition in the health care workplace? Physicians have identified several practical barriers to healthy eating in the work environment. These include lack of time to stop and eat, mostly as a result of staff shortages and workload issues, lack of scheduled breaks, lack of convenient access to food, poor food choices and variety; long distances between work units and catering facilities, and lack of designated places to store food from home. In addition to these practical barriers, physicians have also described how certain attributes of medical professionalism may in fact hinder their workday nutrition (Lemaire et al 2008). For example, doctors have expressed how their strong work ethic and sense of professionalism discourages them from eating and drinking: their feeling was that patient care should come first, or they just needed to get the job done, or that it would seem unprofessional to snack or carry food in patient care areas.

Changing the status quo

Many physicians are aware of healthy nutritional choices and make an effort to eat sensibly while at work. However, given the practical and professional barriers that physicians themselves describe, it is not surprising that they are not always successful. To overcome these barriers, there needs to be advocacy for adequate nutrition in the workplace. Education and dialogue will guide physicians and health care organizations to an increased awareness of the doctors' nutrition patterns, a facilitation of positive change, and an appreciation of the link between physician nutrition and work performance. As physicians and health care organizations promote the benefits of improved nutrition and workplace wellness, everyone will benefit, given the important link between physician wellness and quality of patient care.

Summary

Various personal and workplace factors can make it difficult for physicians to ensure adequate nutrition during their work day. Physicians and health care organizations share a responsibility to improve workplace nutrition by raising awareness, changing nutrition practises and improving access to nutritious food in the workplace.

Case resolution

The resident is facing an issue common to most physicians—difficulty obtaining adequate nutrition during the workday because of a combination of factors that can undermine previously healthy eating habits. The resident becomes more aware of the link between nutrition and well-being. The resident schedules an hour per week outside of work hours to purchase and portion out healthy, well-balanced and portable snacks such as nuts, bagels with cream cheese or peanut butter, fresh and dried fruit, baked rice or whole grain crackers, juice boxes, yogurt and tuna packets. The resident identifies clean and secure storage areas on the units where they work and also keeps a few snacks in their lab coat pocket and locker. The resident makes time for a healthy balanced breakfast daily. The resident introduces a five-minute mid-morning and afternoon snack and hydration break into their operating room and ward work schedule. The resident encourages the other members of the team to do the same. The resident lobbies the health care organization to improve access to and quality of available nutrition, and to provide designated, convenient spaces for nutrition breaks.

Key references

Lemaire J, Wallace JE, Dinsmore K, Roberts D. 2008. *Well Doc? Module 1: Nutrition and Cognition. Report on Interview Data.* Prepared for Alberta Health Services, Calgary, AB.

Winston J, Johnson C, Wilson S. 2008. Barriers to healthy eating by National Health Service (NHS) hospital doctors in the hospital setting: results of a cross-sectional survey. BMC Research Notes. 1: 69.

Introduction: The physician's training

Leslie Flynn, MD MMus CCFP FRCPC

The process of becoming a physician is arduous. It begins for most people with deciding sometime during the undergraduate years of university to pursue studies in medicine. This decision is the first step toward a professional career that is rich in personal rewards and satisfaction. It is also a step that must not be taken lightly, as the years of training are demanding and require self-discipline and dedication. There is a period of intensive preparation, followed by many years of practice, along with continuing education to maintain up-to-date competencies. A commitment to medicine is a commitment to lifelong learning.

Medical school admission

Entrance to medical school is a competitive process. Requirements include an academic record that demonstrates a high grade point average. Applicants are expected to have had a breadth of life experience, as demonstrated in volunteer work, job experiences, extracurricular activities, a proven ability to assume responsibility, an altruistic nature and good interpersonal skills. Most medical schools require applicants to sit the Medical Colleges Admission Test (MCAT). This standardized examination has four sections focusing on physical sciences, biological sciences, verbal reasoning and writing. Paired with these daunting requirements are the financial implications of pursuing medical school admission. There are significant costs to writing the MCAT, applying to medical schools and—if one is successful—medical school tuition. One needs to make a concerted, deliberate choice to pursue medical training.

The medical student

Admission to medical school is a tremendous accomplishment. There is the delight of achievement, the pride of family and friends, and the promise of a rewarding future. The initial euphoria is to be savoured. The memory of this joy will serve successful candidates in good stead during their transition to medical school. This transition is not meant to be easy, but it brings great potential for personal and academic growth. The volume of material to learn is vast and can be intimidating. However, the content all contributes to the fulfillment of a concrete goal—to become a practising physician.

Medical school can present challenges to one's personal life. It may mean a new university, a new living situation, a new city and separation from friends and partners. The personal commitment required can challenge relationships: not everyone will find it easy to accommodate the medical student's new schedule and its demands. Added to these stresses is the financial burden of tuition, which may create or add to an existing debt load.

This combination of challenges tests everyone at some point during medical school. Medical students are at risk of developing unhealthy lifestyle habits. Caffeine, nicotine, alcohol and illicit substances all hold potential for abuse. Healthy eating habits may be eroded. The interests and activities that were once a significant part of life may be neglected or abandoned. All of these factors—poor coping strategies that arise in response to stress and constraints of time—can quickly lead to further difficulties.

It is important to be aware that medical schools have developed a wide range of personal and professional resources to provide support for their students. These resources can be readily accessed through the institution's undergraduate medical education office. The Canadian Medical Association has made financial advice readily accessible to medical students through MD Financial (mdm.ca/students-residents/).

Resident

The term resident originates from bygone days when newly graduated physicians lived within the hospital to further their clinical training and hone their skills. The term lives on, although the times have changed. The resident years—ranging from two to six years in duration—are instrumental for the development of expertise in a chosen specialty. Although many of the same issues that existed in medical school persist, new challenges will come with increased responsibility for patient care, which requires the application of previously acquired knowledge while also expanding one's competency in multiple domains. The intrinsic aspects of a physician's work are those of the resident: the challenge of diagnosis, the interaction with patients and their families, collaborating with colleagues, and the sense of helping to alleviate suffering. It is important to keep these satisfying aspects in the forefront of one's mind, for the daily tasks required in the delivery of this work, paired with the pressures of the health care environment, can lead to doubt and uncertainty. Significant pressures are associated with the training, but developing strategies to ensure that respite is built into one's schedule can help in coping with stress. Trainees are now at a stage in their lives when long-term relationships, marriage and having one's own family may be considered. This is welcome: parental leave is available to resident trainees. All residents need to strive for balance. They need to ensure that they take the vacation and educational leaves that are available to them. They must consciously endeavour to maintain their hobbies and interests. Personal relationships must be cherished and protected. Healthy habits in diet, exercise, and sleep hygiene must be developed. These years will establish a template for the future.

Summary

Becoming a physician requires resilience. Physicians who are satisfied with their career are not only disciplined, effective and productive: they also take pleasure in the work—but not at the expense of leisure, personal and family time. It therefore requires considerable commitment to proactively manage one's life and career. The years of training are preparation for a way of being. It is important for residents to pursue medicine in a fashion that is in keeping with who they are as individuals. What the resident brings to medicine as individuals is, after all, the very reason they were selected.

Key references

Danek J and M Danek. 1997. *Becoming a Physician: A Practical and Creative Guide to Planning a Career in Medicine.* Toronto: John Wiley and Sons.

Goldman LS, Dickstein LJ, Myers M. 2000. *The Handbook of Physician Health: The Essential Guide to Understanding the Health Care Needs of Physicians.* Chicago: American Medical Association.

Sotile WM and MO Sotile. 2002. *The Resilient Physician: Effective Emotional Management for Doctors and Their Medical Organizations.* Chicago: American Medical Association.

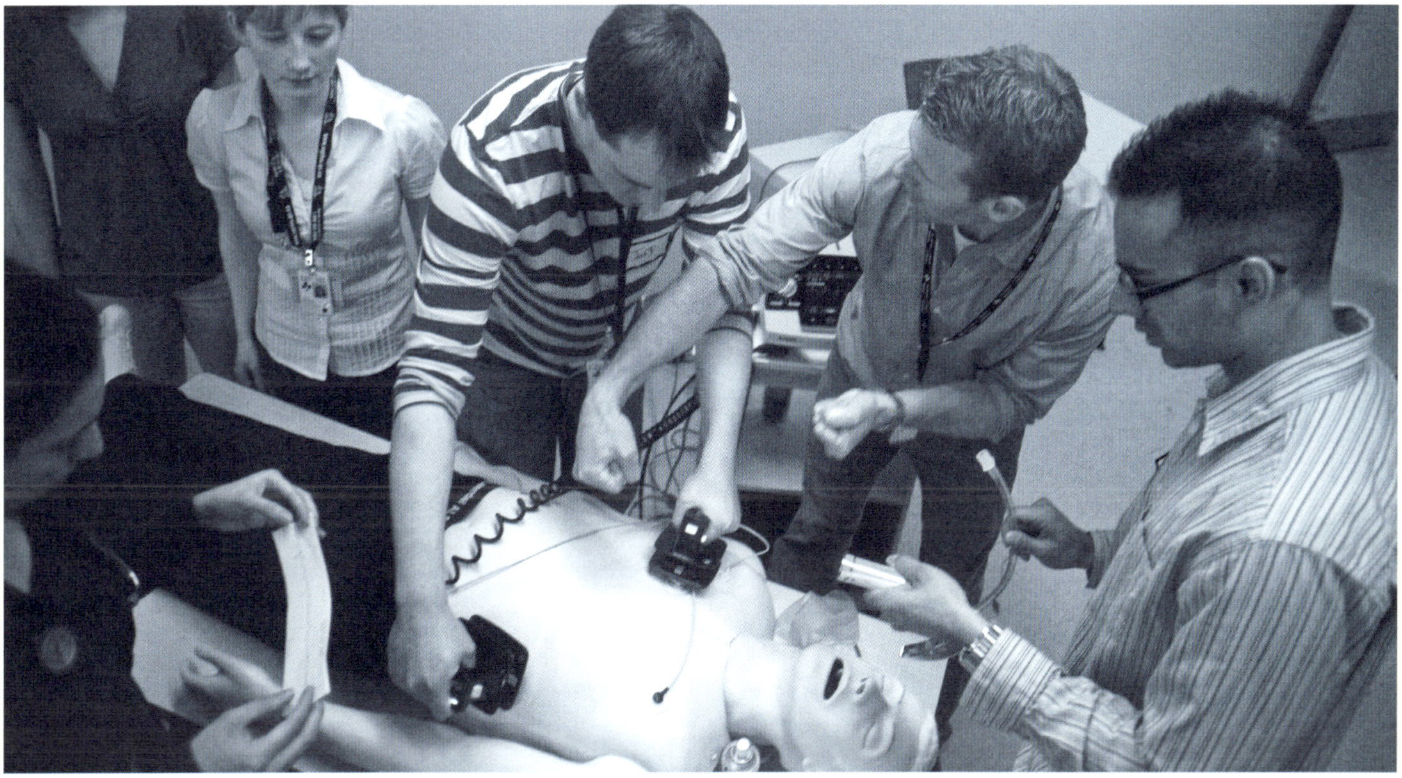

A. Determinants of workplace health

Susan Edwards, MD CCFP FCFP

Objectives

This chapter will

- identify elements of the training environment, both occupational and educational, that affect the well-being of residents,
- describe how these elements can affect the learner both personally and academically, and
- consider ways to improve the training environment to enhance resident resilience.

> **Case**
>
> A fourth-year resident initially identified as a great communicator with a unique ability to make the preoperative patient feel at ease going into surgery, has realized that they have started to dread conversations with patients. Time pressures, negative comments from nursing staff and faculty, highly informed patients with multiple questions, and chronically high case loads are contributing to this dread. The resident has sought feedback from more senior residents and staff who have suggested that it is easier to focus on getting the information needed and move on. The years of on-call are taking their toll, and the resident has heard the surgeons lament that hospital politics will once again mean cutbacks, reduced operating room time and fewer nurses available after hours. The resident is finding that, although they seem to be getting home earlier, the resident is losing the ability to remember details about each patient, is less interested in their stories and, frankly, enjoys their days less. The resident hopes that when they finish residency and start practicing that they might have the inclination and influence to do things differently.

Introduction

Healthy workplaces support their employees in achieving healthy lifestyles, behaviours and adaptive coping skills. They create happier employees, who in turn do better work. Ironically, health care settings can be among the least healthy places to work and learn. Experiences of medical trainees, particularly in their clinical years, can have detrimental effects on their personal well-being, professional behaviours and academic performance. Although residents are generally resilient individuals who cope well with change and uncertainty, they are at risk of the effects of stress, some of which are common to all physicians, and others secondary to their trainee role.

Workplace stressors

Like all members of the health care team, residents experience significant occupational stressors in the course of their usual work. Frequent exposure to suffering and death, acute clinical situations requiring rapid and complex decision-making, prolonged work hours often accompanied by significant sleep deprivation, demanding and increasingly better-informed patients, information and technology overload, social isolation, and fear of litigation are just some of the stressors identified by physicians as affecting their job satisfaction, performance at work and personal well-being. Organizational challenges such as bed shortages and pressures to move patients through the system quickly are stressful for all health care workers but can be overwhelming for residents, who feel that many of these problems affect their ability to do their jobs but are beyond their control.

Additionally, residents are affected by pressures directly related to their role as learners. Acutely aware of the constant need to meet external standards of performance within this intense milieu, residents may feel perpetually under the microscope and fear making errors or bad decisions, or being exposed for their self-perceived imperfection or incompetence. The trainee–supervisor relationship is fraught with challenges ranging from inconsistent evaluation standards, to intergenerational misunderstandings, intimidation and harassment. In a survey of over 1200 residents in the United States, 93 per cent of respondents had experienced maltreatment at some point in their residency; further, they believed this to have significantly affected their performance (Mareiniss 2005). Perpetrators of resident abuse can be faculty but include other residents and health care professionals, as well as patients and their families. In a survey of stress experienced in residency training in Alberta, nurses were identified as the greatest source of intimidation and harassment (Cohen and Patten 2005). Most trainees do not report these incidents, citing fear of academic repercussions.

Residents are not the only recipients of disruptive behaviours. Some report witnessing what they feel are derogatory acts directed at other health care professionals, patients and their families. These incidents can create great dilemmas for residents, who are caught between wanting to be part of the team while not compromising the standards they were encouraged to hold in their formal medical education. Continued exposure to inappropriate behaviour can significantly influence how residents respond to these situations over time; some research evidence suggests that empathy, humanism and compassion decline with advanced years of clinical training.

Teaching resiliency

Although many residents have the sophisticated coping skills that allow them to adapt to the evolving stressors and demands of an emerging medical career, not all enter their training with these abilities. Nor does postgraduate education necessarily support the development of these competencies. The results of immature coping skills range from the temporary crisis in confidence that many residents experience over the course of their training, to mood, anxiety and substance abuse disorders, burnout, potential impairment and, tragically, suicide. Research conducted in the United States has reported rates of burnout as high as 76 per cent among internal medicine residents (Thomas 2004). The idea that physicians can be burned out in a career they have yet to actually start should be of great concern for medical educators. Nor should this concern be limited to the well-being of the trainee. Residents who demonstrate increased unprofessional behaviours are prone to making more medical errors than the average and to providing suboptimal patient care (West and Shanafelt 2007).

The formal postgraduate curriculum on physician self-care and work–life balance is embedded in the CanMEDS Professional Role. Formal curricular offerings on stress management and the development of active coping skills positively influence the well-being of trainees on many levels (Shapiro et al 2000). However, these are frequently not aligned with, or reinforced by, the informal and hidden curricula in which residents learn. Residents are profoundly influenced by the words and actions of the faculty role models they work with every day, (e.g., staff physicians who may be struggling to cope with their own workplace stressors). This informal curriculum, comprised of one-on-one teaching and mentoring moments, appears to have a greater impact on resident learning and behaviour than the formal curriculum (Thomas 2004). Few medical schools have wellness programs to support their faculty, not only in managing their own issues, but also building their capacity to effectively teach these skills to residents. Moreover, organizational challenges and institutional uncertainties shape the systemic aspect of the hidden curriculum, and this also influences resident education. Physicians, who tend not to see themselves as true hospital employees often do not play prominent roles in initiatives for organizational change.

Strategies to promote a healthy working and learning environment for residents need to support the capacity of faculty and health care organizations to improve the culture in which they work. Some faculties of medicine have done just this by developing innovative, bottom-up, relational-centred care and teaching models that are transforming the environment in which all physicians and health care teams function. They emphasize mentorship, communication and compassion, and increased "face time" between residents and faculty in order to promote healthy role modelling and reduce trainee distress (Mareiniss 2005, and Cottingham et al 2008). Training residents to identify and support their colleagues who are in difficulty will also improve workplace health.

Case resolution

The resident struggling with multiple environmental influences that erode job satisfaction. The resident's superior communication skills are waning, and this loss is reinforced by colleagues and faculty. The resident is receiving messages from faculty that suggest there is little control over one's workplace environment. As commonly happens when physicians feel they have limited influence on their work situation, the resident appears to be losing some of the joy and motivation initially brought to training and the resident may be developing a complacency that is threatening their competency.

At this point, the resident needs to reconnect with the core values and beliefs that led to the decision to become a physician. A role model or mentor can have a helpful and significant impact. By sharing their own experiences and by imparting skills of reflective practice, mentors may help the resident recapture the passion and talent for communication. Attending academic half-days on physician self-care or workshops that offer active coping strategies to deal with stress might also resonate with the resident. Regular, informal, small-group discussions with his peers after more formal seminars could offer opportunities for support and advice. Such reconnection will, in turn, foster the development of skills and sustainable practice.

Key references

Cohen JS and S Patten. 2005. Well-being in residency training: a survey examining resident physician satisfaction both within and outside of residency training and mental health in Alberta. *BMC Medical Education*. 5: 21.

Levey RS. 2001. Sources of stress for residents and recommendations for programs to assist them. *Academic Medicine*. 76(2). 142-50.

West CP and TD Shanafelt. 2007. The influence of personal and environmental factors on professionalism in medical education. *BMC Medical Education*. 7 (29).

B. Health and safety

Susan Edwards, MD CCFP FCFP

Objectives

This chapter will

- review the many elements that affect the health and safety of residents in training,
- discuss the multiple policies governing health and safety issues at the university and hospital levels, and
- examine the responsibilities of training programs in educating residents in health and safety issues.

Case

A third-year resident who provides on-call services at a mid-sized community hospital is called to the emergency room to consult on a patient. As the resident returns to the hospital from the portable building where the on-call room is located, the resident reflects on how easily they have adjusted to the increased independence that the staff has entrusted to them on this rotation, and how it has confirmed the resident's confidence in their expanding knowledge and skills.

The triage nurse directs the resident to the room where the patient is waiting and closes the door behind her. The patient is clearly agitated, and the resident's attempt to create a calm interview environment doesn't work. The resident concludes that the environment is no longer safe and gets up to leave the room, at which point the patient blocks the door, shoves the resident, and picks up the chair in front of him with a motion to throw it directly at the resident.

Many minutes later, when the resident manages to calm the patient to the point where the resident can make a safe exit, the resident calls their supervisor at home to review the encounter. Although they discuss the appropriate management plan, at no time does the resident or supervisor discuss the violent incident in detail or talk about reporting strategies, how the resident is feeling, or how they could manage or prevent such risk in the future.

Introduction

Working in health care facilities presents occupational risks to all employees. These include but are not limited to exposures to hazardous materials and communicable pathogens, aggressive and violent patients, and repetitive strain injuries. At the same time, elements of postgraduate training put residents at additional risk of which trainees and their programs or institutions may not be sufficiently aware and so may not adequately address.

Reducing workplace risk

The Royal College's *General Accreditation Standards* state that "all participating sites must take reasonable measures to ensure resident safety at all times." Almost all agreements between provincial resident associations and teaching hospitals clarify the dual status of residents as trainees registered in a university program as well as hospital employees, thereby making the health and safety policies governing both hospitals and universities applicable to those residents. In addition, postgraduate medical education offices have taken steps to develop health and safety policies specifically for their trainees, presumably to delineate appropriate local responses to identified inadequacies or breaches in safety and security.

Health and safety issues fall into the three broad categories of workplace environmental health, occupational health, and personal safety. Environmental health risks include accidents and exposures to hazardous agents such as chemicals and radiation. Occupational risks include exposures to blood and other bodily fluids and to respiratory pathogens. Personal safety risks include exposure to violence perpetrated by patients or others.

To ensure the protection of their residents, postgraduate medical education offices are required to collect immunization data on their trainees and to adhere to a communicable disease policy for residents who have or present a risk of transmissible disease. In addition, programs traditionally offer orientation in working safely with hazardous materials and in communicable disease precautions and protocols. Individual programs that involve specific and frequent environmental exposures (e.g., radiology, radiation oncology, pathology) provide more focused training to minimize risks of special relevance to these residents. Because most residents are briefed on safety issues during the first week of training when they may already feel overwhelmed and have a limited capacity to absorb new information, a real understanding of how to respond to a safety issue might not be acquired until the first time a resident experiences it directly, for example through a needle stick injury.

A further challenge of preparing residents to protect their own safety is that some risks are not immediately apparent, or may simply be accepted as an unavoidable part of the job. Many of these are related to the number of hours spent in the health care setting, very often at the least secure times. On-call residents and their nursing colleagues are frequently in the position of being on the front line, often in the emergency room setting. This, combined with their relative inexperience in identifying when a situation is getting out of hand, can increase their risk of assault by a patient. While psychiatry residents may be at particular risk given the profile of their patient population (36-

64% of residents among various studies), Canadian data suggest other residents experience similar rates of patient assault (40% of internal medicine residents) (Waddell et al 2005).

These incidents can be extremely stressful to residents, who may feel inadequately trained to deal with them on their own and may be unfamiliar with reporting protocols. Accreditation visits routinely examine the physical layout where residents train to ensure they are properly equipped, for example by means of alarms and proximity to support staff, to prevent violent assaults by patients. However, these assessments might not examine other less controllable settings were residents see patients, such as community clinics and patients' homes. Residents perpetually balance the fear of putting themselves or a patient at risk with a reluctance to reveal their vulnerability by requesting help from staff.

Where specific education and training programs exist to manage workplace violence, residents and students are more likely to report incidents and get the support they need. Postgraduate programs should equip their residents with the skills to identify high-risk situations, to de-escalate potentially violent encounters, to respond urgently to a violent situation, and to proceed with a formal reporting strategy that includes reviewing, documenting and debriefing the incident.

Other personal safety issues include safe and secure access to call rooms and transportation to and from work sites (e.g., security escort to cars after dark). Intimidation and harassment by faculty, staff and colleagues can present safety risks that residents are, generally speaking, reluctant to disclose. In addition, excessive fatigue from long work hours can affect judgment and reaction times, leading to increased risk of needle stick injuries, adverse events, medical error and motor vehicle accidents.

Summary

Residents are aware that certain risks are associated with the work they do. Some of these risks might not be acknowledged as presenting potential dangers; others might be accepted as part of the job. Whether from a sense of duty, not wanting to miss out on a great learning opportunity, or fear of repercussion if they appear too hesitant or dependant, residents may overlook health and safety issues as an essential component of their education. Training programs need to identify health and safety breaches as prime teaching opportunities and to ensure that residents are trained in risk assessment and in policies and procedures to follow when breaches occur.

Case resolution

Like many mid-level residents, this resident is trying to balance the confidence gained from working more independently with the limitations of their experience. Residents may not consider that they will be placed in situations that could cause them harm, and therefore rely on hospital policies and procedures to ensure their safety needs are met. In this case, such procedures were flawed. The resident was focused on making a proper diagnosis and management plan, rather than on assessing the risk of the situation. The resident began the patient encounter without considering the state of the patient, the layout of the room, whether there was an appropriate response system if they were in danger (e.g., security personnel, alarm system), or whether the patient had the means in the room to injure the resident. Additionally, the resident may not have had the skills and training to calm an increasingly agitated patient, and did not have a supervisor present to review the situation beforehand, or to help the resident when the situation got out of hand.

After the incident, no formal procedures of how to report, document and review the incident were followed. The resident and emergency room staff were not appropriately debriefed, and therefore the opportunity for residents, faculty and the institutional administration to learn from this event was lost.

An additional risk for this resident was inherent in the location of the call room in a portable building outside the main hospital where the resident could have been isolated from any security back-up, and from which the resident was required to travel in the dark to get to the work site.

Key references

Cloverdale JH, Louie AK, Weiss Roberts L. 2005. Protecting the safety of medical students and residents [editorial]. *Academic Psychiatry*. 29: 329–30.

Moscovitch A, Chaimowitz GA, Patterson PGR. 1990. Trainee safety in psychiatric units and facilities: The position of the Canadian Psychiatric Association. *Canadian Journal of Psychiatry*. 35: 634–5.

Waddell AE, Katz MR, Lofchy J, Bradley J. 2005. A pilot survey of patient-initiated assaults on medical students during clinical clerkship. *Academic Psychiatry*. 29: 350–3.

C. Work hours: Coping with residency training

Derek Puddester, MD MEd FRCPC

Objectives

This chapter will:

- describe the implications of residency work hours for quality of education and patient care and safety, and
- summarize strategies for the management of work hours that can have a positive impact on learner and patient outcomes.

Case

One of the nurses has made a complaint about a senior resident's level of irritability, and another is questioning whether the resident is practising safely: apparently, the resident made two dose related errors while on call. The resident requests a meeting with the program director, who notes they look exhausted. The resident indicates that all the residents are exhausted. The resident explains that they are working maximum call; a number of residents are on parental leave, leaving little flexibility in the system; handover typically drags on until the early afternoon; educational demands continue unabated (with the residents primarily teaching each other topics as part of their preparation for certification examination); and a bus strike has contributed to lengthy commutes. The resident feels they are doing what they can to demonstrate their abilities as a resident but admits to being exhausted. In fact, the resident produces a letter from their physician stating they require three days off work for health reasons.

Introduction

Hours Watch (www.hourswatch.org), a collaborative of the Committee of Interns and Residents of the United States and the American Medical Student Association, have collated a number of scientific studies that show the following results:

On-call shifts of 24 consecutive hours or more are associated with

- a sevenfold increase in the incidence of preventable medical errors,
- a 35 per cent increase in the risk of committing a serious medical error,
- a 61 per cent increase in the risk of accidental percutaneous injury,
- decreased performance on tests of response and vigilance,
- double the risk of having a motor vehicle accident during the post-call commute, and
- performance impairment similar to that induced by a blood alcohol level of 0.05 per cent.

They also report that

- shorter work hours improve patient care,
- shorter work hours are associated with decreased mortality among high-risk patients, and
- in spite of evidence showing the value of reduced work hours for trainees, many institutions and trainees resist efforts to create safer work schedules.

In different parts of the world, including our own, health and education systems have struggled with the issue of resident work hours. In Canada, we have typically negotiated work hours on a provincial/territorial basis, in keeping with the fundamental structure of our health care system. Throughout Europe and the United States, considerable attention has been paid to resident work hours on a larger scale; this has had the benefit of bringing increased awareness of and attention to patient safety and outcome management from the perspective of health professional fatigue.

Potential solutions

Respect collective agreements. Because training systems and trainees alike can ignore the boundaries set by a collective agreement, the challenge is to create a culture of dual accountability and respect to ensure adherence. Particularly areas of workplace safety such as fatigue management, collective agreements can be helpful only if they are respected.

Embrace a safety culture. Embedding safety as a core workplace and educational value can have a positive and sustainable influence if it is genuine, explicit and promoted. If all members of the health care team come to embrace safety issues honestly, then the adoption and promotion of the principles of fatigue management will readily evolve.

Standardized handover. Handover is a particularly vulnerable time for errors in patient care. Written and oral handover practices that are interdisciplinary and team-oriented have been shown to reduce such errors. In addition, handover is increasingly being recognized as a skill that requires formal training, evaluation and revision. At times, this critical period in patient care has been used to resist evolution in residency education and training; however, the real issue is one of opportunity for improved quality outcomes in the area of patient handover.

Encourage and reward scheduling innovation. Work-hour reductions in the United States and Europe have been associated with unusual and innovative practices. Using shift-work models familiar in the world of emergency medicine but less so elsewhere, some surgical programs have eliminated the need for call. Increased dedication to interdisciplinary care, increased recognition of the skills of other professionals and new professionals, and new models of operating health systems after hours have earned awards on both sides of the pond.

Tame the pager. Increasingly, programs are developing policies to minimize the use of pagers. Empowerment of other health professionals, the use of text messaging, and increased training in the appropriate role and scope of paging has been associated with improvements in efficiency, learning and sustainability.

Invest in other human resources. By optimizing the involvement of physician assistants, nurse practitioners, phlebotomists, procedure teams and other health professionals, health systems that are straining to deliver quality care with limited human resources can eliminate transferable tasks from a resident's workload, such that many of the more common aspects of care are attended to with no critical loss of educational opportunity to the trainee. These professionals can help ensure that the needs of patients are met without the unnecessary reliance on exhausted, and potentially dangerous, trainees at the bedside.

Free transportation post-call. Exhausted residents (and indeed, all hospital professionals) are particularly vulnerable to accidents after they leave the hospital post-call. For a small investment in transportation that safely allows residents to reach home post-call, hospital systems could make a significant difference in health and sustainability.

Accessible education. Residents who stay post-call for educational sessions learn little, and the loss of opportunity for rest places them at risk of accident and error. By developing e-learning at every opportunity (e.g., uploading videos of lectures and rounds, capturing teaching sessions on podcasts, maintaining a database of slide presentations and associated hand-outs, and considering what ongoing learning can be delivered through online courses) residents can be enabled to take advantage of learning opportunities when they are alert, motivated and able to concentrate.

Many other practical and comprehensive solutions to the burden of excessive work hours during residency, as described by Ulmer and colleagues can be considered in a Canadian context. As we continue to improve patient safety, quality outcomes and excellence in residency training and education, we will need to be open to more systemic interventions targeting fatigue management.

Case resolution

The program director immediately approves the leave request. She then alerts the departmental chair of the human resource issues that, she readily admits, are more severe than had been realized. New on-call protocols are implemented that reduce overall work hours for the remaining residents, a systemic process for handover is implemented, and a small number of physician assistants and nurse practitioners are hired permanently. The program director also begins to shift educational sessions to models that allow for ready digitization and remote access by residents.

Key references

Barger LK, Ayas NT, Cade BE, Cronin JW, Rosner B, Speizer FE, Czeisler CA. 2006. Impact of extended-duration shifts on medical errors, adverse events, and attentional failures. *PloS Medicine*. 3 (12):3497.

Barger LK, Cade BE, Ayas NT, Cronin JW, Rosner B, Speizer FE, Czeisler CA; Harvard Work Hours, Health, and Safety Group. 2005. Extended work shifts and the risk of motor vehicle crashes among interns. *New England Journal of Medicine*. 352 (2): 125–34.

Shetty KD and J Bhattacharya. 2007. Changes in hospital mortality associated with residency work-hour regulations. *Annals of Internal Medicine*. 147 (2): 73–80.

Ulmer C, Wolman, D M, Johns MME, eds. 2009. *Resident Duty Hours: Enhancing Sleep, Supervision, and Safety*. Washington (DC): National Academies Press.

D. Professionalism: Reasonable expectations

Richard Cruess, OC MD FRCSC and Sylvia Cruess, MD CPSQ

Objectives

This chapter will

- examine how the reasonable expectations of residents or physicians may conflict with those of their training program, the profession, individual patients or society,
- consider how to manage expectations on the part of patients, residents and practising physicians, and
- discuss how to establish priorities to provide excellent patient care while maintaining a balanced and healthy life.

> **Case**
>
> A final-year surgical resident has been the lead doctor treating a 62-year-old widow with carcinoma of the colon. The resident carried out the surgical procedure with the assistance of the attending surgeon. The patient trusts the resident and regards the resident as her surgeon. The patient is aware of the diagnosis and understands that some treatment decisions must be made. She lives alone and wants her family to participate in the discussion about treatment options before her discharge. The family members must travel from their home at a distance so the only time when this discussion can take place is at 7 p.m. The resident has been on call since the night before, is required by the residents' contract to be off-duty, and the family has tickets to a hockey game with their son as a birthday treat.

Introduction

Professionalism has been described as the basis of medicine's social contract with society. The profession and its individual members are granted the privilege of autonomy in practice, a monopoly over the practice of medicine through licensure, the right to physician-led regulation, and both financial and nonfinancial rewards. In return, physicians are expected to place patients' needs above their own, to assure their own competence and the competence of their colleagues through regulatory processes, to demonstrate morality and integrity, to address issues of societal concern, and to be devoted to the public good. This "bargain" with society leads to tangible expectations on the part of patients and society on one side and on the part of physicians and the profession on the other. Striving to meet all of the obligations expected of physicians in a complex and frequently underfunded and understaffed health care system often places impossible demands on individual physicians.

Managing expectations

Patient's expectations have been well documented and are generally reasonable. First and foremost, they expect that their physician will be competent. They wish to be listened to, to be treated with compassion, to be able to trust their physician, to have their needs placed above that of their doctor, to have a physician who is present for them and accountable, and to have their personal autonomy respected.

Physicians also have expectations of their patients. They expect to be trusted because it is difficult to carry out the healing function in the absence of trust. They wish to be given sufficient autonomy to exercise their professional judgment. They expect patients to accept some responsibility for their own health. Canadian physicians want their health care system to be equitable, adequately funded and staffed, and to afford reasonable professional freedom. They expect to lead a life in which there is a balance between the practice of medicine, family and other interests. Finally, they expect reasonable rewards, both financial and nonfinancial.

For their part, residents must cope with the expectations of their mentors, the institution within which they work, and their training program. In Canada, the broad outline of these expectations is documented in a contract. However, residents frequently feel pressure to go beyond their contractual obligations. Indeed, there are times when a professional must. For example, it is inconceivable that a resident would leave a care setting at the end of a shift when to do so would put a patient's life at risk. However, one of the major objectives of limiting time on call is to protect the health of the resident, ultimately for the sake of patients—it is well documented that the judgment of a tired or overstressed resident or physician can be impaired.

Although it can be difficult at times to meet the legitimate expectations of patients and society, most of these expectations are relatively uncontroversial. The most significant tension that may arise stems from a conflict between altruism—a sense of obligation to put patients' needs above one's own—and the physician's need and desire for a balanced lifestyle. In contemporary Canada, this tension is exacerbated by a real shortage of physicians and other health care professionals, which has led to tremendous pressure on physicians, including residents, to see more patients. No one likes to see others go without access to a physician or endure long waits for treatment. Thus, each resident and practising physician constantly balances the needs of individual patients and of society with their own personal well-being.

There is also the potential for tension between loyalty to one's fellow residents or practitioners and the public's expectation that the profession will assure the competence of its members. Physician-led regulation requires each individual physician to accept responsibility for the competence and behaviour of his or her colleagues. A resident who is aware of unprofessional or unethical conduct on the part of another resident or practitioner must take appropriate action. It is the responsibility of the training program to have well-publicized processes to allow this to occur, both for the sake of patient safety and to establish a pattern of appropriate responses on the part of the resident. It is essential that these processes ensure that no harm to the resident's career follows from the disclosure of unacceptable conduct on the part of others.

The process of becoming a medical professional occurs gradually throughout undergraduate education and postgraduate training and continues throughout professional life. It is a process of socialization during which individuals begin as uninitiated members of the lay public and gradually acquire the culture of the medical profession. This happens in parallel with the transformation from non-expert to expert clinician. In recognition of this, there are different expectations for physicians in training depending on the level they have attained. This is true not only in terms of the acquisition of knowledge and skills, but also with respect to the social contract. As students and residents accept increasing levels of responsibility for patient care, they are expected to gain a more sophisticated understanding of their professional responsibilities and their obligations to patients and society. The resident in the case study is in his final year of training and will presumably be in practice very shortly. For that reason, more is expected of him by both the training program and the patient than would be true of a medical student or first-year resident.

It is important that residents in training understand that the issues involved are fundamental to medicine's relationship to patients and society, that they are able to analyze the various situations that arise, and that they can make the often difficult personal choices required. They must be able to decide when they must defer their own needs, and when maintaining personal well-being requires that they fall short of the expectations of their program or their patients. Training programs bear a heavy responsibility in ensuring that unreasonable demands are not chronically imposed upon residents, and that tensions concerning professional versus personal priorities are discussed openly throughout a resident's training. Behavioural patterns that are detrimental to a healthy lifestyle are often set during residency training. This must not be allowed to happen. On a more positive note, being aware of the tensions that inevitably arise in practice, and having an opportunity to reflect on them in a supportive environment, can help to establish patterns of behaviour that both preserve the professionalism of medicine and lead to healthy patterns of living.

Case resolution

Many issues in medicine have no satisfactory solution. One must often look for the "least-worst" path in trying to meet the legitimate expectations of one's patients and one's self. For a professional, the interests of a worried and vulnerable patient must come first. However, if the resident in this case example stays to meet with the family, they will violate the terms of the resident contract and disappoint their own family.

Possible solutions are rescheduling the meeting, which will be difficult; enlisting the help of the attending surgeon, who has the primary fiduciary responsibility in this case; or missing or arriving late at the hockey game, in which case members of the resident's family will be asked to make a personal sacrifice in deference to the resident's professional priorities. There are times when one's responsibility to patients must take precedence over family needs or contractual obligations. Compromise is certainly acceptable on occasion, and for good reason. However, if "duty first" becomes a pattern of behaviour, the health of the physician and personal relationships may suffer. This issue must be addressed openly during training. Respected role models play an important part in helping each individual resident understand the importance of the issues and the fact that limits must be placed on the expectations of all parties to the social contract.

Key references

ABIM Foundation American Board of Internal Medicine, ACP-ASIM Foundation American College of Physicians–American Society of Internal Medicine, European Federation of Internal Medicine. 2002. Medical professionalism in the new millennium: a physician charter. *Annals of Internal Medicine.* 136: 243–6.

Cruess RL and SR Cruess. 2008. Expectations and obligations: professionalism and medicine's social contract with society. *Perspectives in Biology and Medicine.* 51: 579–98.

E. Work hours: Coping with professional duties

Jason R. Frank, MD MA(Ed) FRCPC

Objectives

This chapter will

- discuss the challenges presented by long duty hours in medicine, and
- describe strategies for coping with the risk of fatigue to protect physician health, patient safety and sustainable practice.

> **Case**
>
> A first-year resident feels life is like a runaway train. They feel tired and irritable all the time, and their world is overflowing with medicine (facts, patients, readings, rounds, procedures, test results, assignments and call). The resident misses their family, cooking a good meal, and having time to read something unrelated to medicine. They can't remember their last workout. The resident could use a good night of sleep, too, but they are on call again tonight and know that is not going to happen. The resident is starting to find patients and their complaints annoying. When they observe their supervisor they are working with today, the resident notices the supervisor looks just as tired. The resident wonders if they are cut out for medicine.

Introduction

That medical practice is characterized by intense and long work hours is an understatement. Patients do not choose the hour they become ill, and twenty-first century medicine is a 24/7/365 enterprise. Physician shortages, an aging population, and difficulties accessing health care mean that the patients physicians see have increasingly complex needs and are sicker. The exponential growth in medical knowledge and technology also place greater demands on physicians, and physicians-in-training, than ever before. It is easy to understand why many clinicians have difficulty dealing with their professional workload.

Physicians tend to work more hours than the average in a population. In the 2007 Canadian National Physician Survey, the mean reported time spent on professional duties, before call, was about 51 hours per week across all specialties, practices and ages. Sixty-one percent of physicians also reported working 30 additional hours on call per week, and 10% reported working 60 hours on call per week. Physicians-in-training, with a few short years to prepare for practice, typically spend 60, 80 or more hours on duty every week, depending on the specialty and the jurisdiction. These long hours of duty put physicians at risk for a number of negative consequences.

> **Factors that contribute to physician fatigue**
>
> Fatigue = individual characteristics × nature of the work × work hours × time of day × work setting / breaks

The impact of long duty hours

Working around the clock can be socially, physically and psychologically challenging. Long duty hours can lead to isolation from friends and support networks, straining relationships and preventing physicians from maintaining former activities and connections. Extensive time at work can tax one's energy and lead to irritability, depressed mood, substance abuse and other mental health problems. Prolonged and extensive duty hours around the clock are a risk factor for weight gain, immune dysfunction, infertility, diabetes, gastrointestinal complaints and coronary artery disease. In fact, in their health effects, extreme duty hours such as years of shiftwork involving night shifts and sleep loss have been equated with smoking a pack of cigarettes per day. Working outside of regular business hours, as in doing call or shiftwork, disrupts the circadian rhythms critical to well-being. This can lead to cumulative fatigue, burnout and medical error.

Work hours and fatigue

Traditionally, fatigue was thought to be a simple equation: fatigue = hours of work. Now, it is understood that the work that fatigues one person one day might not have the same impact on someone else, or even on the same person in other circumstances. Fatigue is perhaps better thought of as a function of an interaction of different factors (see textbox): the individual (e.g., sleep status, other health factors, coping strategies, skill level), the nature of the work (e.g., intensity, interruptions, ergonomics), the hours on task and opportunities for breaks (e.g., naps, meals, pauses), time of day (days, evening, nights), and the work setting (e.g., safety, familiarity) (Frank and Ovens 2002). In turn, fatigue can lead to neurocognitive deficits at work, and this can lead to inattention or medical error, putting patients at risk (Crosskerry 2008). Over the longer term, physician fatigue can lead to mental or physical health problems, burnout, and exit from practice.

Strategies to cope with long work hours

What can a physician do to mitigate the effects of long work hours? Barring radical changes in residency education, the numbers of physicians, and cures for diseases, medicine will continue to involve long hours of intense activity for most members of the profession. However, the five general strategies described below can support healthy work habits, counteract the effects of fatigue, promote safe practice, and avert burnout (see chapter 11-E).

Maintain rhythms. Maintaining physiological, social and psychological rhythms is key to preventing fatigue, illness and burnout. Circadian rhythms have a profound impact on our physiology, and so their disruption should be avoided wherever possible. Good sleep hygiene can help address the impact of working after regular business hours. Similarly, it is important for physicians to maintain their social and psychological rhythms, including time with family and friends. Attendance at key family events should be fiercely guarded, for example. Thinking about a regular ebb and flow to the days of the week, even when weekend work is required, is helpful in preserving a sense of well-being. Finally, a regular exercise routine not only enhances physical fitness but also promotes quality sleep, cognitive function and stress tolerance.

Counteract fatigue. Among the many techniques for counteracting fatigue, the most important by far is to sleep when one is tired. However, long duty hours can preclude this. Other techniques include the judicious use of caffeine, avoiding other drugs such as alcohol, taking breaks and naps, finding ways to de-stress, exercising, and working in bright light.

Manage time effectively. Although one might learn a good deal about time management during medical education and training, few programs take this issue seriously enough to make a substantial impact on physician health and effectiveness. The good news is that a wealth of advice is available for those who seriously want to acquire good time management techniques. The key competencies are knowing oneself, prioritizing and setting goals, following a plan, getting organized, and leveraging resources. Becoming personally effective requires insight into one's priorities, strengths, weaknesses and values. Only then can one set priorities in alignment with one's fundamental goals. Techniques to assist prioritizing include values clarification, writing a personal mission and vision statement, and imagining one's legacy or biography.

Time and energy are precious resources, and allocating them effectively takes skill. Techniques in this domain include setting personal and professional goals (short-, medium- and long-term) and using a personal organizer (e.g., MS Outlook software or a Blackberry) for daily, weekly, monthly, and yearly calendar management. Focus is achieved by critically appraising and aligning decisions with one's values and mission in life, and saying "no" to some tasks. Setting priorities allows activities to be realigned with goals. The key is to make a plan and stick to it as much as possible, while revisiting the plan frequently. To-do lists, a continuing professional development plan, or a career trajectory are examples of roadmaps to success. To get the most out of these priorities, a well-organized work space and filing system, clear workflow processes, and the avoidance of distractions are essential. Finally, it is important to manage available resources, whether assistants, colleagues, mentors, or technologies. Effective time management is a critical domain of medical ability, and not only allows a physician to be more productive but also assists with the ability to balance professional and personal needs and demands.

Engage others. The value of dialogue with other key individuals is often overlooked in discussions about physician work hours. It is important that, individually and as a profession, we ensure that others understand the nature of our work. Loved ones can become frustrated by our frequent absences, and others in our lives may need to be educated about the demands on our time. More broadly, decision-makers in society need to be aware of the nature of medical work to ensure that health care polices and resource allocations promote sustainable practices for all health professionals.

Revitalize. Renewal and revitalization are a final essential ingredient. Physician culture, with its dedication to work and responsibility, can make it difficult to take holidays. Vacation time should be planned and taken; it is wise to ensure that the next vacation is booked by the time the current vacation is done. All professionals need time to de-stress and reflect on their career and priorities, to renew their energies, and to focus on personal priorities outside of medicine. These strategies are essential to preventing burnout and ensuring success and longevity.

Case resolution

The resident decides to talk to a staff member they respect about this fatigue. They have a great conversation, and the resident feels hopeful. The resident decides to take the weekend off medicine, spend some quality time with their family, have a run, and see a movie. The resident will also take some time to reflect on how they organize their week to see if they can "work smarter." The resident signs up for a Time Management for Physicians workshop and decides to drop one of the roles they play in the residency program to focus on things that are most important to their personal well-being and career.

Key references

College of Family Physicians of Canada, Canadian Medical Association, Royal College of Physicians and Surgeons of Canada. 2007. *National Physician Survey.*

Frank J, Ovens H. 2002. Shiftwork and emergency medical practice. *Canadian Journal of Emergency Medicine.* 4 (6): 421–8.

Crosskerry P. 2008. Shiftwork, fatigue, and safety in emergency medicine. In Croskerry P et al, eds. *Patient Safety in Emergency Medicine.* New York: Lippincott.

F. Intimidation and harassment in training

Jordan Cohen, MD FRCPC

Objectives

This chapter will

- discuss the elements of intimidation and harassment and how they affect residents during training, and
- describe an approach to dealing with intimidation and harassment within the context of a residency program.

> **Case**
>
> Your residency program is under accreditation next year. (1) As a faculty administrator, what is one activity that you will institute as a faculty administrator to prepare for this event? (2) As a resident body, what process could you undertake to prepare for accreditation?

Introduction

Intimidation, harassment and workplace bullying have probably existed as long as the institution of medicine, but have started to be addressed by medical faculties only within the last two decades. At a fundamental level, intimidation and harassment are defined not only by the behaviour and motivations of the perpetrator, but by the response of the individual who is targeted. It should be seen as causing a negative effect on the victim (e.g., stress). Although no instance of intimidation or harassment is ever appropriate, such acts must be persistent to be deemed "bullying." Many academic administrators will not feel enabled to act on an allegation of intimidation and/or harassment unless there is clear documentation of the event, identification of the individuals involved, and a demonstration that this was not a single occurrence. This highlights the importance of reporting such events, not only so that medical trainees can protect themselves, but also to help prevent their recurrence against others. By taking action against bullying behaviours, medical students and resident can help to change the culture of medicine for the future.

Where intimidation and harassment leads

Intimidation and/or harassment can lead to poor job satisfaction and psychological distress. It has been associated with mental health problems and a desire to leave medical training. It significantly influences physician health, retention and, ultimately, patient care.

Where intimidation and harassment occur

Physicians in training experience intimidation and/or harassment in all areas of medical training—that is, in the clinical, research, administrative and political realms. More than half of respondents to a recent Canadian survey reported that they had experienced intimidation and/or harassment while in residency training. Training status and gender were felt to be the two main bases for the intimidation and/or harassment. The abuse was reported to have originated from nursing staff as well as teaching faculty and to have occurred most often in the form of verbal abuse. Other forms of intimidation and harassment reported by resident physicians have included inappropriate physical contact, sexual harassment, the assignment of work as a punishment, loss of privileges and opportunities, and recrimination for reporting unacceptable behaviour.

Dealing with intimidation and harassment

For intimidation and harassment to be tackled effectively, it is essential that trainees have a safe and efficient mechanism to deal with these behaviours. In some cases, it is faculty who may be more concerned about the repercussions of reporting for their trainees, who for their part may have a naive faith that the reporting process is adequate and accessible. On the flip side, trainees should recognize that, in many cases, the individuals involved in bullying are not aware of the effect they are having. In many cases, individuals who intimidate and/or harass others need education in effective communication as teachers and administrators, rather than disciplinary action. Most medical schools have now adopted directors or deans of equity to deal with conflict issues between faculty and trainees. Many of these individuals directly report to the dean of medicine or to "high-level" faculty committees with the ability to institute change. They focus on the content, psychological issues and procedures surrounding the issue of conflict.

The Royal College of Physicians and Surgeons of Canada requires that adequate mechanisms be in place to deal with issues of conflict during residency training, including intimidation and harassment. Program directors, faculty members and residents must be aware of these resources and deem them to be effective in dealing with such concerns. Programs that are unable to demonstrate such mechanisms may be put on probation and risk losing their accreditation status.

In tying such importance to this issue, the Royal College ensures that programs will endeavour to create a training environment that limits intimidation and harassment, adequately deals with issues that arise, and takes steps against the perpetuation of unacceptable behaviours, for the benefit of future generations of medical trainees.

Key references

Cohen JS, Leung Y, Fahey M, Hoyt L, Sinha R, Cailler L, Ramchandar K, Martin J, Patten S. 2008. The happy docs study: a Canadian Association of Internes and Residents well-being survey examining resident physician health and satisfaction within and outside of residency training in Canada. *BMC Research Notes*. 1: 105.

Paice E, Aitken M, Houghton A, Firth-Cozens J. 2004. Bullying among doctors in training: cross sectional questionnaire survey. *BMJ*. 329: 658–9.

Case resolution

The residency program directors should ensure that all teaching faculty are aware of policy and procedures for dealing with intimidation and harassment (e.g., by distributing a flow chart). A meeting could be organized with the primary faculty and the director of equity for your school to educate them on appropriate actions to take when dealing with issues of conflict with trainees.

Residents should also be clear on the policy and procedures. This may be done with a teaching session using case examples or role playing from the director of equity. Residents should also be encouraged not to conceal, but rather report concerns around intimidation and harassment so that the accreditation team can make appropriate recommendations that will ultimately be addressed by the individual programs.

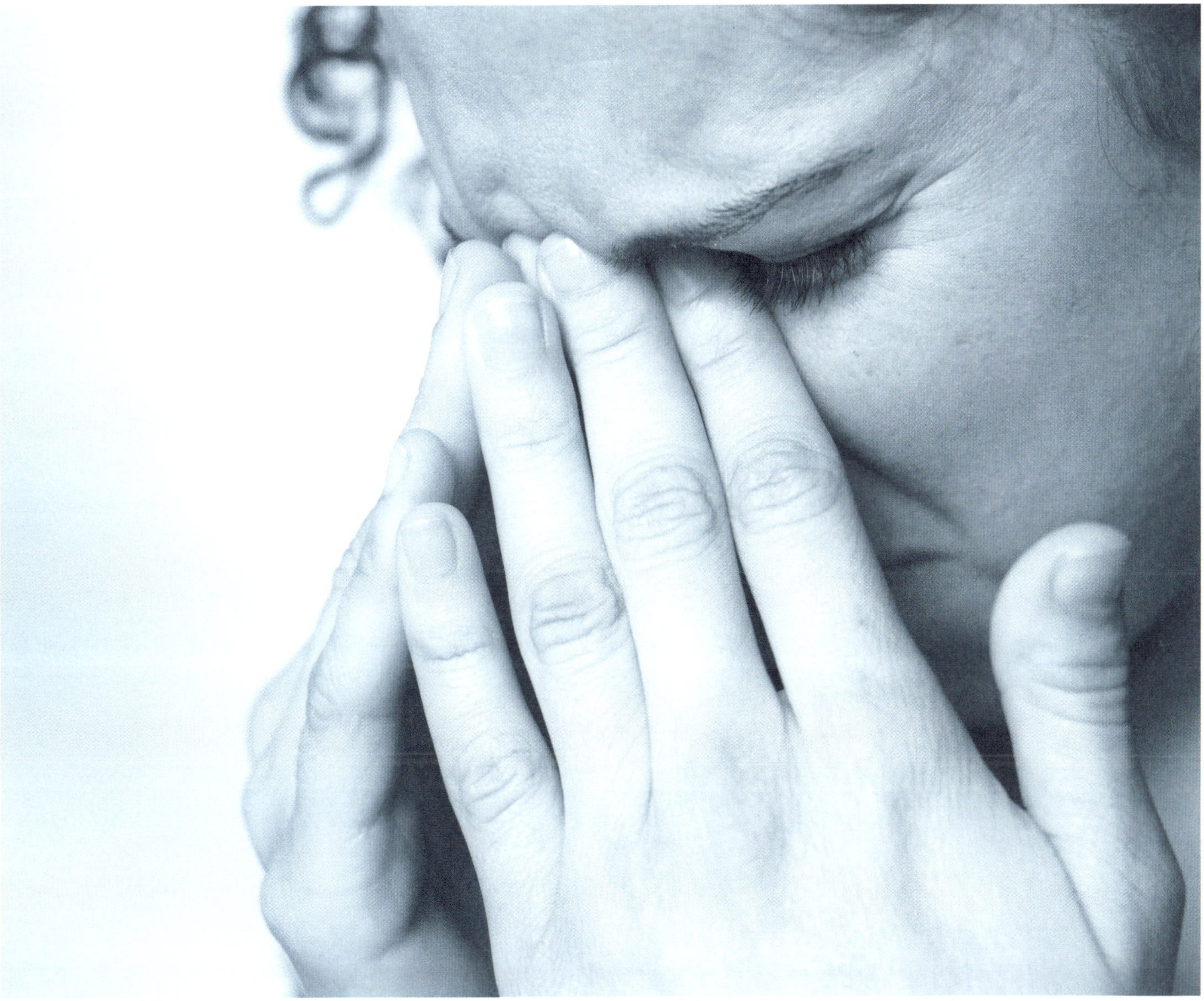

Introduction: Collegiality

Jordan Cohen, MD FRCPC

Collegiality essentially refers to the cohesiveness and solidarity of a group founded in a commitment to a common goal. Collegiality involves certain rights and is tempered by specific obligations. In academic contexts, it pertains to a commitment to the maintenance, support, exchange and dissemination of knowledge. Collegiality allows physicians to educate one another on clinical matters, to pursue scholarly objectives and, ultimately, to support one another in their lifelong professional development. Physicians have an obligation to put restrictions on their collegiality: in particular, they must give the welfare of their patients priority over their collegial relationships.

Although collegiality is highly prized by individual practitioners and medical administrators, it is not always explicitly taught. All of the CanMEDS Roles embody the attribute of collegiality. One cannot become an effective Scholar and Medical Expert without sharing information with peers. One cannot be an effective Health Advocate without the cooperation of one's supervisors and peers—which will itself be shaped by the degree of collegiality that exists among them. One learns effective approaches through the wisdom and example of other practitioners. The physician's role as Manager requires (especially nowadays, when relationships between physicians and other members of the health care team are less hierarchical than in the past) a sense of trust and empathy among members: in other words, a sense of collegiality. To fulfill the obligations of their Professional Role with respect to patient care, ethical behaviour and self-regulation, physicians cannot function in a vacuum. In addition to supporting these domains of competency, collegiality by definition engenders the kind of mutual respect and support that helps to prevent the intimidation and harassment of colleagues. Moreover, where healthy collegiality exists, physicians will not only support one another during good times, but will also protect one another's health by recognizing when colleagues are in trouble and helping them to get the support they need.

Collegiality in medical environments fosters efficiency, improved physician health and, in the case of academic institutions, a high output of scholarship and innovation. Medical departments that do not foster collegiality suffer from poor communication among colleagues, resulting in decreased productivity, health problems, burnout and staff attrition. Collegiality is an important predictor of job satisfaction, and efforts to increase collegiality often increase morale.

The following sections consider how physicians can support one another as colleagues. Challenges to collegiality are discussed with respect to disruptive physician behaviours, conflict management, and gender-based and generational tensions. Finally, relationships between physicians and all professionals on the health care team are discussed.

Teaching strategies

Resident leaders, medical educators and program directors should all endeavour to foster collegiality in professional relationships. One method of doing so is to encourage the mentoring of residents by faculty members, and of medical students by residents, whether in person, by email or through websites. Within a training program, topics on medical collegiality can be discussed among peers at scholarly events (e.g., during academic half-days), between supervisors and residents, and between residents and program directors. As a body, residents can decide on a topic concerning physician health that could be mediated by increased collegial relations (e.g., emotional stress related to time pressures in training) and invite a faculty member who feels comfortable sharing personal experience to facilitate a discussion group.

Evaluation strategy

Although collegiality can be measured by teachers through general observation, more formal methods include a 360 degree evaluation process by which residents are evaluated by all members of the health care team, including their peers. Peer feedback is often perceived as less critical and constructive in criticism, when discussing topics of communication with colleagues. This kind of evaluation process can ensure that the resident is evaluated fairly by all members of the team and removes pressure off of the physician preceptor who may have challenges providing critical feedback. For the residents involved, it builds skills in giving feedback on professional matters to peers.

Key reference

Frank JR, ed. 2005. *The CanMEDS 2005 Physician Competency Framework. Better Standards. Better Physicians. Better Care.* Ottawa: The Royal College of Physicians and Surgeons of Canada.

Mangiardi JR and ED Pellegrino. 1992. Collegiality: What is it? *Bulletin of the New York Academy of Medicine.* 68 (2): 292–6.

A. Supporting one's colleagues

Paul A. Farnan, MB BCh FCFPC

Objectives

This chapter will

- apply the concept of collegiality to an academic setting, and
- discuss the broader responsibilities associated with collegiality, especially with regard to physician colleagues.

Case

Although a second-year resident has been an important innovator and leader among their peers, over the past three months they appear to have become more withdrawn and isolated. A formerly vibrant personality seems to have been replaced by moodiness and introversion. The resident's spouse of eight years was, most unusually, absent from the recent department dinner, and there are rumours of marital difficulties. Some of the resident's peers notice the resident drinking more alcohol than usual one night before driving home. There are also rumours that the resident may have been in some sort of trouble with the law recently. In addition, a legal proceeding involving one of the resident's cases, which had an adverse outcome two years ago, is scheduled in civil court soon.

Introduction

Like college and colleagues, the word collegiality derives from the Latin *collegere*: to read together. Collegiality, in an academic setting, is often thought of in association with the concept of a collegium: "a collection, body, or society of persons engaged in common pursuits, or having common duties and interests, and sometimes, by charter, peculiar rights and privileges."

When a collegial atmosphere exists in an academic centre it can create a safe and productive setting for both teachers and learners. Collegiality can create a culture in which uncertainty, lack of knowledge and feelings of incompetence are both tolerated and discussed. It maximizes open communication and the dissemination of ideas and information. In such a setting, a collegial faculty would be one that values a commitment to the sharing of knowledge.

Cultivating collegiality

The importance of the social setting of learning is well recognized. For example, learning can be facilitated by group activities such as workshops and tutorials. When well organized, these activities expose each learner to a range of beliefs and attitudes and allow for the sharing of views and opinions. By serving both to broaden perspectives and foster the mutual respect of both, teacher and learner, this approach can also provide an important model for maintaining respect within the physician–patient relationship. By fostering collegiality, academic medicine has the opportunity to enhance the quality of medical graduates as well as, to provide a good basis for future learning.

Collegiality is not limited to academic settings. Medicine is practised in a health care system that is constantly changing and increasingly demanding. The importance of teamwork and effective communication to the delivery of quality medical care is well recognized, and the term collegiality has come to refer to professionals working together as equals and sharing in decision-making. Care of the patient can be a complex challenge that requires the skills of a range of health care professionals. In speaking of multidisciplinary care, we can forget that such care involves more than a multidisciplinary group comprised of physicians. True collegiality involves collaboration with other health care disciplines, and there is much that each can learn from the others. In fact, the reality is that team members need one another in order to form a resilient and sustainable workforce. Having said that, collegiality between collaborators is not automatic. It needs to be fostered and nurtured with respectfulness and a mature desire to work together productively and supportively.

Collegiality offers the benefit of a safe and protective community that can help us to cope in the face of stressful work environments. However, collegiality is more than a camaraderie or advantaged club: it implies certain duties and responsibilities. Society does not appreciate a self-protective collegiality that circles the wagons around questionable professional behaviour, or that ignores the obvious deterioration of a colleague's performance to the detriment of patient safety. And so it is important to remember that, like everyone else, physicians get sick and grow old, and that in the process their competence can be compromised. As is discussed elsewhere in this handbook, certain aspects of the culture of medicine, together with typical attributes that otherwise hold physicians in good stead, can make physicians reluctant to admit when they find themselves in difficulty. However, the physician's responsibility to maintain his or her own health in order to practise safely also extends to a collegial duty to be aware of the health and fitness of others. This is not always easy.

Collegial support becomes particularly important when we are ill and lose insight into our own professional performance. In the past, ill physicians, worried that their medical licence might be put in jeopardy, remained silent until a complaint was reported to a regulatory body or an adverse event occurred. Meanwhile, their colleagues would refrain from intervening. Even now, despite the availability of organized physician health programs in every Canadian province to assist physicians in difficulty, we cannot ignore our collegial responsibility to support one another other at the local level. Neither should we wait until problems are of such severity that regulatory bodies need to be involved. Workplaces should have mechanisms in place to ensure that potentially impaired practitioners promptly cease practice until their fitness to practise can be assessed. This is what true collegiality at a community level is all about. Too often, however, a misguided sense of collegiality makes physicians hesitate to respond to a colleague in difficulty or encourages them to cover up and effectively enable impaired or substandard professional performance.

An organized and responsible method for dealing with matters of potential physician impairment would involve early identification of physicians who might require assistance and the provision of timely and caring intervention when it is needed. Help could include offering encouragement, covering practice duties, referral to remedial assistance and, eventually, mentorship for physicians returning to work after an absence. It is to be hoped that incapacitated colleagues will respond appropriately to support and advice, but at the end of the day we cannot ignore our legal and ethical obligations to report to the appropriate bodies impaired physicians who insist on practising despite reasonable offers of assistance.

Summary

A supportive collegial group works proactively as a team to ensure the optimal function of all members. It is not focused only on the individual practitioner's health, but also on the health and well-being of the group, as a whole. Such a group works not only at identifying organizational problems that contribute to the stress of health care staff, but also encourages a healthy and respectful workplace. These collegial activities would typically involve preventive or proactive initiatives aimed at minimizing negative workplace stressors in order to promote a healthy and sustainable work force.

Case resolution

It is important for any organization or group to cultivate collegiality and mentorship. In this case, rumours are circulating and presumptions are being made, but no one knows if there is any real basis for them. The resident might have a substance use disorder, a significant depression, an adjustment disorder or some other reason for the apparent change in behaviour. It is certainly not appropriate to stand by and do nothing. Nor is it a colleague's role to try to diagnose or to treat the resident. It is appropriate, however, for a trusted colleague or colleagues to respectfully ask to meet with the resident privately and to present their genuine concerns about the behaviours that have been witnessed. It would be appropriate to offer assistance in connecting the resident with a personal physician if the resident doesn't have one.

In this case it would be appropriate for the colleague or colleagues to research contact information for the local physician health program and assist the resident in organizing an appointment with medical staff there. It might even be fitting for a colleague to accompany the resident to such an appointment, but not to be part of that meeting. Alternatively, it might be appropriate to follow up with the resident to try to ensure that they had indeed made contact with a resource. Academic departments or group practices should cultivate a resource list of primary care physicians who are community based and not necessarily associated with academic departments. These providers should have experience in caring for physician colleagues and medical families, recognizing the sensitive nature of the doctor-patient relationship with a doctor patient (or family member).

Key references

Brown G, Rohin M, Manogue M. Culture, collegiality, and collaborative learning. In Sweet J, S Huttly, and I Taylor, eds. 2003. *Effective Learning & Teaching in Medical, Dental & Veterinary Education*. London: Kogan Page. pp. 18–35.

Mangiardi JR and ED Pellegrino. 1992. Collegiality: What is it? *Bulletin of the New York Academy of Medicine*. 68 (2): 292–6.

B. Conflict management

Paul A. Farnan, MB BCh FCFPC

Objectives

This chapter will

- examine the assumptions that are often made in the characterization of conflict,
- describe factors that influence styles of dealing with conflict, and
- discuss collaborative attitudes and communication skills that support the creative resolution of conflict.

> **Case**
>
> Two enthusiastic and ambitious residents seem to have butted heads regularly on several issues during their three years together in residency. Conflicts occur repeatedly, whether it surrounds organizing the on-call rota, holiday schedules, or topics for grand rounds. The conflict seems to be escalating, and each sees the other's behaviour as stubborn and inflexible. As is typical of unresolved conflict, the situation is becoming personalized, and both now see the other party as the main problem, rather than whatever issues it was that originally led to the conflict. The situation is becoming difficult for the department as a whole, as both residents each seek to recruit colleagues into their camp.

Introduction

The term conflict often conjures images of violence, as in the conflict of war. In this module we focus on interpersonal conflict, which occurs when human need or interest is frustrated. It has been defined as "a situation in which one or both persons in a relationship are experiencing difficulty in working or living with each other. This usually occurs due to different or incompatible needs, goals or styles" (Fisher 1977). Interpersonal conflict is a natural by-product of change and growth and arises in any developing relationship. People who have healthy interpersonal relationships do not have conflict-free relationships. Rather, they accept the inevitability of conflict and succeed in identifying tensions early and resolving them. They also have insight into how their own history influences how they see conflict and respond to it. They are conscious of their personal communication techniques and are aware that conflict makes constructive communication difficult. Because these facets of conflict resolution are so complex, a better designation might be conflict management, since not all conflict ends up being resolved.

Sources of conflict

More than ever before, health care is a complex and rapidly changing field that relies on teamwork. Although conflict in medical workplaces and academic settings is common, it can be difficult to deal with, especially when its determinants are poorly understood. Given that interpersonal conflict is potentially all around us, it is important to learn strategies that help us to manage it, whether it involves colleagues, partners, spouses or others.

Most instances of conflict appear to have had an immediate, observable trigger, a hot-button issue of some kind. In reality, the problem is usually more complex. There are typically many other variables, of which the parties involved might not be fully aware. Such variables include the power relationships, true needs as opposed to apparent wants, and styles in dealing with conflict. When we are involved in an interpersonal conflict it is important to be aware of our own typical responses to conflict—our "conflict styles." This involves cultivating the honest self-awareness that allows us to be conscious of the lenses or filters through which we see the world. It is normal to make presumptions and assumptions on the basis of experience. But these beliefs are not always true. If we can honestly appreciate and understand how we see the world, we can begin to perceive our own biases and, ultimately, to gain insight into why we are in conflict.

When we are in conflict we can demonstrate behaviour that is either defensive or open. A defensive style is usually more adversarial, and reflects the extent to which we are attempting to satisfy our own needs. An open style is one of cooperativeness, and reflects the extent to which we are willing to satisfy the other person's needs.

Kenneth W. Thomas and Ralph H. Kilmann described five modes of dealing with conflict-handling styles, which can be characterized in terms of their relative position along the two axes of behaviour mentioned above (e.g., assertiveness versus cooperativeness). They are: competing (forcing), accommodating (smoothing), avoiding (withdrawing), collaborating (problem-solving) and compromising (sharing). All behaviour can make sense when you understand the other person's unmet needs. In order to appreciate somebody's needs we need to set an environment of trust and honesty. In addition, we need to listen actively and explore what it is they are truly seeking.

Given that so many factors influence our personal behaviour in conflict it is wise to remember that when in conflict it really is "all about me," rather than the other person. It is worth asking oneself the question, "why am *I* in conflict?"

Communication

One cannot discuss conflict without considering communication. Our dealings with other people depend on how we interact or communicate with them. Communication has always been vital to our continued existence—it allows us to meet our basic needs for survival and safety and permits our inclusion in social groups. Although we might use the same language or words when we communicate, we don't necessarily use them in the same way. Meanings are not inherent in words. Rather, meanings are intrinsic to the interpretation of those words. Communication involves what is heard or otherwise perceived, and not merely what is said. Tone of voice, gestures, body language, timing, context, and so forth, all influence what is "heard." The problem with non-verbal signals is that they are often unintentional—and may be more likely to convey our true meaning than our words are. Communication is dynamic because, particularly in a conversation, we send and receive information at the same time. Moreover, communication is irreversible—once the message is sent, we might be able to retract it, but we cannot un-say it.

When emotions are involved, such as in times of conflict, the inherent difficulty of communication increases. Conversations involving conflict are likely to foster defensiveness and a misreading of messages, and have an unfortunate potential for misunderstanding. If we are to communicate effectively during an interpersonal conflict, it is important to remove the emotional charge from the situation.

Working at effective communication leads to better understanding between people and reduces judgmental assumptions. We must work to appreciate how the other individual sees the issue that has prompted the conflict, rather than inflexibly insisting on how we think they should see it. Conflict resolution requires a genuine desire to understand. It involves a commitment to engage in problem-solving with the other party, and requires ground rules that permit open exchange and reduces the need for defensiveness. Fortunately, resisting the urge to respond defensively is a skill that can be learned. Viewing the conflict as a problem to be solved mutually so that both parties feel that they are benefiting from the resolution is the goal of collaborative conflict management. No relationship can be long-lasting and rewarding without conflict management. At the end of the day it is worth bearing in mind that the relationship is as important, if not more important, than the outcome of the particular conflict at hand.

Case resolution

This conflict could have been addressed at an earlier stage, before it became so damaging. Both residents have been oblivious to the ways in which they have each contributed to the ongoing conflict. Each has viewed the other as the problem, rather than looking at shared problems that they might have solved collaboratively. They have reached the point where they are unable to communicate because the conflict is so emotionally charged.

The department head decides to organize a conflict management workshop for all faculty and residents. This helps everyone gain a better understanding of the nature of interpersonal conflict, and stresses the importance for the collegiality of the department of addressing conflict proactively. The facilitator then works privately with both residents to help them appreciate the importance of learning conflict management skills as part of their training. He helps them to examine their engrained approaches to conflict, the life experiences that have shaped their conflict styles, and their tendency to make inaccurate assumptions about each other. He reminds them of the importance of trust, coaching them on a process of active listening that uses a non-confrontational vocabulary. He advised that parties in conflict should speak of:

- **Observations.** Stick to what you personally experienced: "I'm noticing that..."
- **Thoughts.** Describe conclusions that you drew from what you saw or heard: "I'm thinking that..."
- **Feelings.** Sharing your feelings to allow others to have greater empathy: "I'm feeling..."
- **Needs.** Expressing needs doesn't blame or assign fault. It simply states what would help or please us: "It would be helpful for me... What would work for me is..." (McKay et al 1995)

Key references

Lindahl K and A Schnapper. 2002. *The Sacred Art of Listening: Forty Reflections for Cultivating a Spiritual Practice.* Vermont: Skylight Paths Publishing.

Rosenberg MB. 2003. *Nonviolent Communication: A Language of Life.* Encinitas (CA): PuddleDancer Press.

Stone D, Patton B, Heen S. 2000. *Difficult Conversations: How to Discuss What Matters Most.* London: Penguin Books.

C. Disruptive professional behaviours

Paul A. Farnan, MB BCh FCFPC

Objectives

This chapter will

- review examples of and define disruptive professional behaviour, as well as its impact on health care organizations and training/learning environments,
- explore the personal characteristics as well as the elements of organizational cultures that can influence physician behaviour, and
- consider how to develop a consistent and timely systemic response to situations involving disruptive behaviour.

> **Case**
>
> The chief resident in internal medicine has arranged to speak to the program director about one of the PGY3 residents. The chief is "fed up." This resident is irresponsible. The resident doesn't come to teaching sessions, doesn't show up for clinics on time, is always late when showing up for on-call responsibilities and therefore never receives appropriate handover regarding the patients. The other residents are complaining to the chief. The nurses on the ward and the emergency room staff have started calling the chief whenever this resident is on call. The chief wants something to be done.

Introduction

The term "disruptive doctor" is often thought of in relation to physicians who demonstrate a pattern of offensive or objectionable behaviour, such as berating staff in front of patients or using intimidation tactics when supervising residents. Other types of disruptive behaviour, such as late or inappropriate responses to pages and calls, being chronically late, or not showing up for meetings, may attract less attention, but can be equally problematic by undermining teamwork.

Many definitions have been developed to describe disruptive behaviour. The College of Physicians and Surgeons of Ontario defines it as follows: "Disruptive behaviour is demonstrated when inappropriate conduct, whether in words or action, interferes with, or has the potential to interfere with, quality health care delivery."

Effects on patient care

Disruptive behaviour has negative consequences both for the delivery of patient care and for the smooth running of medical departments. It can lead to a higher incidence of medical error and other adverse events, and has the potential to stifle the respectful collaboration and interdisciplinary collegiality that are crucial to effective care delivery in today's complex health care environment.

Disruptive behaviour also has negative effects on medical learning environments—it models inappropriate behaviours for students and residents, impedes their ability to acquire clinical skills, and damages the collaborative culture necessary for learning.

It is estimated that three to five per cent of physicians demonstrate a pattern of behaviour that could be described as disruptive. It is not unusual for these physicians to be highly skilled technically, to be busy experts in their field, and to be champions for their patients. They commonly see themselves as superior to others in their clinical competence and insist that others submit to their way of doing things. In addition, they often lack insight into the impact of their behaviour on others.

Causes

There is no single cause of disruptive behaviour. Although it is not generally associated with substance use disorders, other underlying physician health issues such as stress and burnout can be contributing factors. Disruptive behaviour has been associated with certain personality characteristics such as obsessive-compulsive or narcissistic traits; however, it is dangerous to assume that disruptive behaviour always betrays a personality disorder. It is often a result of an inability to deal with the conflict inevitable in the face of stressful work environments and rapid change. Indeed, disruptive behaviour can be a sign of failure within a system, where conflict has become personalized and poor leadership prevails.

Responding to disruptive behaviour

Health care organizations typically have no formal process for dealing with disruptive behaviours, even when they have had to react to incidents in the past. The focus is often exclusively on the individual's behaviour, to the exclusion of any examination of external influences. But focusing solely on changing the physician's behaviour is not productive. It is also vital to examine systemic factors in, and responses to, disruptive behaviour.

For too long, physicians as a group have assumed that the issue of professionalism is covered adequately in medical school. But is it clear that physicians themselves must show leadership in addressing disruptive behaviour in their practice settings and academic departments. The issue should be approached even-handedly, taking logical steps. First, what constitutes disruptive behaviour needs to be clearly defined and its impact understood. Guidelines for approaching disruptive behaviour need to be developed and distributed to all key stakeholders. The development of a professional code of conduct to address workplace interpersonal behaviour is also important.

Sotile and Sotile suggest a simple example of such a code that could be easily implemented by any medical staff organization or department. It states:

> "To satisfy our mission, all members of the medical and health staff will treat patients, staff and fellow physicians in a dignified manner that conveys respect for the abilities of each other and a willingness to work as a team. Behaviour that is deemed to be disruptive to promoting an atmosphere of collegiality, cooperation, and professionalism will not be tolerated."

Although one might feel that formalizing such a code of conduct should be unnecessary, it is vital to be able to refer to such a code when the need to manage a problem involving disruptive behaviour arises. Such a code has a preventative role as well; it can help create a culture of respect and collegiality by offering guiding principles for all who work in the institution. The code should be consistent with the philosophy of the larger organization, or could be the same code used by all providers in the organization.

Even with an agreed-upon code of conduct, it can often appear that nothing is done in response to episodes of disruptive behaviour. Therefore, a clearly defined set of policies and procedures that everyone is familiar with should also be developed. Like the code of conduct, these policies and procedures should be formulated with input from all stakeholders. They need to be developed through consultation and consensus; to be credible, this should involve the "grass roots." Overarching principles to be followed consistently during the development process would include fairness, objectivity, transparency, confidentiality and timeliness. The resulting policies and procedures should establish which individuals will be involved in the various stages of the process—from accepting and reviewing reports, to notifying and meeting the physician exhibiting the problem behaviour, arranging assessment if necessary, defining resolution and reconciliation goals, setting return-to-work expectations, and monitoring conduct after assessment or treatment.

After the policies and procedures have been developed, it is critical that managers, physician leaders and new department heads are briefed on their elements and implementation. Ensuring that orientation to the code of conduct and policies and procedures occurs on receipt of hospital privileges or employment can prevent problems down the road.

It should be stressed that if administrative physicians were to hurriedly write a unilateral code of conduct or policies and procedures manual while in the midst of a disruptive behaviour crisis, this action would likely be perceived as punitive and as personal and thus be doomed to failure. The time to write such guidelines is before a problem occurs.

Case resolution

When the chief resident becomes aware of a resident who is not meeting their responsibilities, the chief confirms the facts and meets with the resident to notify them of the concern and discuss the issue. The chief obtains a commitment that the behaviour will not be repeated. The chief then follows up to monitor future behaviour knowing that future trangressions will need to be brought to the program director's attention. The program director must ensure there is a policy or guidelines on the expectations about professional responsibility.

Lastly, in establishing realistic re-entry expectations and conduct boundaries for physicians returning to the workplace after a conflict arising from disruptive behaviour, it is wise to involve the physician concerned. This may also be a good time to review the organization's code of conduct, policies and procedures, to ensure that the physician returning is clear on the expectations placed on them. After a return to work, consistent monitoring and reinforcement of appropriate behaviours will be critical to ensuring that change is lasting.

Summary

The appropriate approach to this issue should be one of rehabilitation and support rather than punishment. As a first step, organizations need to clarify their definition of disruptive professional behaviour. Leaders must appreciate what contributes to and provokes disruptive behaviour so that educational and training programs can be implemented to decrease the likelihood of its occurrence and to improve overall effectiveness of communication among health care teams.

Every organization should be prepared to deal with disruptive conduct by establishing clear, unambiguous and carefully crafted policies and procedures that are specifically designed to address such behaviour. It is no longer acceptable to rely on the "professionalism" lectures that were provided early in training or to assume that the physician involved "should know better." Leaders should review their current policies relating to disruptive behaviour, where such policies already exist, and obtain commitment from stakeholders and leaders within the organization to develop or revise policies as needed. The medical staff organization will usually need the support and collaboration of the medical administration to ensure that there is a cooperative joint effort. At the end of the day, an approach to disruptive behaviour that is fair, consistent, timely and understood by all within the organization should be the goal.

Key reference

Sotile WM, Sotile MO. 2002. *The Resilient Physician: Effective Emotional Management for Doctors and Their Medical Organizations.* Chicago: American Medical Association.

D. Generational issues in contemporary medicine

Leah J. Dickstein, MD MA DLFAPA and Derek Puddester, MD MEd FRCPC

Objectives

This chapter will

- describe key differences between generation Y, generation X, the boomer generation, and the traditionalist generation, and
- identify key areas in which generational differences can contribute to conflict, and consider the unique opportunities presented by today's generational mix for the practice of medicine in Canada.

Case

A mid-career physician in a busy academic hospital enjoys working with residents and values the unique perspectives and energies they bring to clinical and academic work. However, the physician is increasingly concerned by what feels like a slippage of professional duty, commitment and formality. On rounds, the physician expressed dissatisfaction with a medical student who was playing with her phone, a resident who was not wearing a tie, and a fellow who indicated he needed to leave by 5 o'clock to pick his daughter up for a soccer game. All three trainees, in turn, made a complaint about this behaviour to the site director for education.

Introduction

The Canadian medical community embraces a diverse mix of learners and practitioners. This diversity has many facets, including gender, race, cultural heritage, political alliance and philosophical world view. One facet of diversity that is becoming increasingly relevant to educational programs is that of generation. Obviously, any framework that clusters diverse people into specific categories is at risk of overgeneralizing; however, the following sketches of today's generations and their traits may be a useful way to conceptualize challenges that arise in training and practice environments.

Generation Y. This cohort generally consists of the population born from the early 1980s to the early 2000s. Also known as the millennial generation and the "net" generation, this cohort came of age in a time of political stability, economic advantage and particular encouragement and support. They embrace digital communication and are skilled multi-taskers who are not insulted when someone does a Google search on their iPhone in mid-conversation, responds to an urgent text message during small group learning, or accesses the latest clinical information through their Blackberry. Finally, they are often image-driven, favour self-expression over self-control, and have a skeptical view of traditional models of authority, power and hierarchy. They work hard to get a job done but do so in a highly flexible manner and on their own terms.

Generation X. Born between roughly 1960 and 1980, this cohort is also known as the "Me Generation" and the "Lost Generation." They are the first generation to grow up in a culture of medicare and in a workplace influenced by residents' associations. Gen X also came to age in an era of instability in Canadian medicine, when a lack of professional unity contributed to tensions around billing number restrictions, loss of training flexibility, and early-career decision-making. As a result, they are wary of medical structures and institutions, protective of their own career paths, and motivated by careers that facilitate their personal and professional balance. They will work hard, but demand negotiation, respect and clarity in order to protect the balance between their personal and professional lives.

Baby boomers. Born roughly between 1940 and 1960, the Boomer cohort is highly focused on professional success and competition, productivity and output, and respect for traditional hierarchy and roles. Known to roll up their sleeves and pitch in, they are more prone to sacrifice themselves to realize the goals of their institution. Their rates of burnout are high (up to 42 per cent in Canada), as are their rates of divorce or separation (52 per cent).

Traditionalists. Born generally before the mid-1940s, this senior cohort of physicians has a wealth of experience and talent. Many have now retired from active practice but have had a profound and valuable influence on traditional structures in medicine, including practice standards, training methodology and professionalism.

Sources of tension

The varying experiences and expectations of these generational cohorts can give rise to misunderstandings and tensions arising from different working styles and apparent values. Sources of this tension can be described as follows.

Perspectives on work/life balance. Boomers and Gen X/Y seem to be most at risk of conflict in this area, as their perspectives are often very different. Regardless of the nature of the differences, they must be respected. Boomers need to facilitate learning and practice environments that sustain learners while preparing them for the rigours of practice. This is not a particularly easy task and requires careful mentoring, graduated responsibility, respect for boundaries/limits, and acknowledgement of collective agreements and respectful interpersonal communication.

Use and engagement with technology. Multi-tasking is often viewed with disdain by Boomers, particularly when they witness learners communicating with more than one person at the same time (e.g., sending a text message to a peer while listening to a lecture). Aspects of multi-tasking require open discussion and dialogue, as well as flexibility: the X and Y generations are often able to safely divide their attention across multiple domains and do so with no intention of disrespect or disregard.

Informality and individuality. The shift in contemporary culture away from hierarchical expectations in social relationships is notable. Respect from others no longer follows automatically from a position of authority; rather, it is earned and managed on the basis of relationships. Younger generations need to be sensitive to the culture of their more senior colleagues, while Boomers and traditionalists will gain points by demonstrating principles of equity, respect and autonomy. In addition, younger cohorts need to be reminded, often through role modelling, of how to project a professional stance through dress, language and tone appropriate to each situation.

Health care human resource needs. There is a dramatic shortage of physicians in Canada, and many Gen Xers (and, very soon, Gen Ys) will soon be moving into leadership positions in education and practice. In the past, Boomers and traditionalists earned such positions after "paying their dues," learning on the job and having time to develop readiness for leadership. More than ever before, younger generations need mentorship and support from more experienced colleagues as they take on heavy responsibilities early in their career.

Now is not the time for any generation to be dismissive of another. In fact, intergenerational diversity brings with it a remarkable opportunity to integrate and synergize perspectives and to create new synergies and energies within the practice of medicine.

Messages for the learning and practice environment

When managing or preventing the many conflicts that can arise in an intergenerational training or practice environment, it can be helpful to recognize basic wants and needs that apply to every generation. In general, people simply want to be:

- respected, by being given meaningful work, being treated fairly and with dignity, having the opportunity to earn loyalty and trust, and having control over one's destiny;
- recognized through the monetary and non-monetary acknowledgement of effort, achievement and innovation;
- remembered as having made a valued contribution during their time in an environment;
- mentored in a supportive, non-judgmental fashion to achieve their best, manage their weaknesses, gain insight into their own nature and progress to the next phase of their career;
- consulted on any decisions that will affect them in a manner that acknowledges that their ideas may be part of a solution rather than part of a problem; and
- connected to their peers, supervisors, families, significant others,communities and their inner selves in a meaningful and genuine way.

With flexibility, a sense of humour, honesty and transparency, all generations can readily engage one another to solve almost any challenge they face.

Case resolution

The physician attended a seminar on intergenerational opportunities and realized that many of the behaviours interpreted as disrespectful were, in fact, the opposite. The physician began to ask learners about the content of the multi-tasking efforts and enjoyed hearing about the information and knowledge they so easily accessed and integrated into their knowledge set. The physician also reflected on the healthy boundaries the students set between personal and professional life and the physician began to make changes in their own practice in order to spend time with family and significant others. Finally, the physician purchased a smartphone and, after a tutorial with a medical student, found that it improved efficiency remarkably. The more open and flexible the physician became, the more trainees began to come for mentorship and guidance.

Key references

Smith W. 2008. *Generational Differences: Fact, Fiction ... or Should We Just Get Back to Work?* New York (NY): Deloitte Development.

Puddester D, Gray C, Robertson C. 2005. Training generation x: A theme of growing importance. *Royal College Outlook* 2:1 Spring; 8–10.

E. Interdisciplinary relationships

Janet Wright, MD BSc(Pharm) FRCPC

Objectives

This chapter will

- describe how good relationships with all members of the health care team can improve patient safety, reduce the incidence of burnout and improve work satisfaction;
- describe factors that influence working relationships with other health care professionals, peers and faculty; and
- identify steps that can be taken to improve collegiality.

> **Case**
>
> A first-year resident working in a major urban hospital is five months pregnant when she does her rotation and finds that the nurses are very kind to her. She spends long hours talking with them while on call and feels that she has an excellent relationship with the nursing staff. One night while she is on call a woman in labour begins to show signs of fetal distress. The resident asks the nurse to change the woman's position, to get an IV bag so she can start an IV, and to call the obstetrics fellow. The nurse looks at her and leaves the room without responding. The resident changes the patient's position and stays with her. The nurse returns with the fellow and starts to explain the patient's situation. The fellow notes that she is in the appropriate position and agrees with starting an IV, at which point the nurse runs to get it. The resident is astonished that the nurse ignored her request and yet is willing to run to obtain things for the fellow. She wonders what she could have done differently in her relationship with the nurse and feels angry that her requests were ignored.

Introduction

The culture of health care has changed over the past few decades from one in which physicians are clearly in charge to a culture in which physicians are part of a multidisciplinary, interprofessional team. Well-functioning teams have great potential in delivering excellent patient care and improving patient safety. Poorly functioning teams, particularly those with communication problems, can present significant risks to patients. The ability to establish collegial relationships with members of the health care team is essential.

Physicians must not only work with other health professionals in a collegial fashion but must also establish good relationships with clinicians and faculty members in other specialties. Collegiality enables academic interchange and collaboration at the level of the individual case, in the development of new techniques for medical care, and in research activities, improving outcomes in all of these spheres.

Collegial relationships

Two common themes in the literature of professional collaboration and collegiality in health care are a shared purpose in caring for patients and the ability to treat others with integrity and respect. The American College of Physicians manual states:

> "Physicians share their commitment to care for all ill persons with a broad team of health professionals. The team's ability to care effectively for the patient depends on the ability of individual persons to treat each other with integrity, honesty and respect. Particular attention must be paid to certain types of relationships and power imbalances [...] such as attending physician and resident, resident and medical student or physician and nurse (ACP)."

Murray Goldstein states this idea more simply "[c]ollegiality requires a fostering of the attitude 'we are in this together'."

Benefits to collegial relationships

The advantages of good relationships among members of a health care team are well documented in the literature. Among the benefits are improved care to patients and improved patient safety. The open sharing of information, and the attitude that questioning and checking is expected, leads to safer care. It is crucial for a pharmacist to call and point out a medication error or a nurse, acting on previous experience with a patient, to question an order for a medication to which she believes the patient is allergic. Patients also report improved satisfaction with care when members of the team work together.

Both physicians and nurses who work on well-functioning teams report improved work satisfaction, less burnout, improved morale, increased motivation and reduced conflict. Jensen and colleagues have identified supportive relationships, characterized by positive personal relationships, effective professional relationships and good communication with consultants and other members of the multidisciplinary team, as one of the most significant factors in improving the resilience of physicians.

What makes collegial relationships difficult?

Given the many benefits of collegiality, it is important to address potential barriers to good working relationships. Bulgar and Bulgar highlight problems that subspecialists encounter in relating to their generalist colleagues. For their part, family physicians frequently point to disparaging comments made about them by specialist colleagues. We forget that it is impossible if not futile to expect one physician to acquire a good working knowledge of all parts of medicine at all times. It can also be difficult to be respectful of others when service demands are high, time is short, and we are fatigued from being on call.
Other members of the health care team can have overlapping

areas of expertise and scopes of practice; this can feel threatening to physicians who are not confident of their role on the team or who may have a different approach to a problem. We are often ignorant of the knowledge and skill in other disciplines because we are not educated or trained together. This can lead to so-called "turf wars." The CMA policy on achieving patient-centred collaborative care stresses the need to clarify roles and scopes of practice as well as lines of accountability and responsibility. In an exploration of professional relationships between nurses and physicians, Zelek and Phillips found that many nurses and physicians still overtly and covertly resist the equalization of power that true teamwork requires. Salvage and Smith argue that while assertive nurses resent being put down by doctors, physicians resent being challenged by nurses.

Improving interprofessional collegiality

It is only common sense that treating others with respect will improve relationships and improve team communication and effectiveness. Achieving this, however, can be more complicated than it sounds. In a study of interprofessional collaboration within intensive care units, Lingaard and colleagues showed that levels of collaboration or conflict within the ICU team and with other specialties fluctuated on the bases of six key catalysts: authority, education, patient needs, knowledge, resources and time. They identified two dominant mechanisms at work in team functioning:

1. **The perception of ownership:** this can include perceived ownership of specialized knowledge, technical skills, equipment, clinical territory and even the patient himself or herself. For example, a nurse described her frustration when residents rely on her assessment but when presenting at rounds make it sound as if they have done the assessment themselves.
2. **Process of trade:** there is an ongoing process of trade going on in all interactions. Trade can be in concrete physical commodities such as equipment and beds, but it also includes abstract social commodities such as respect, goodwill and knowledge. For nursing groups the most dominant currency for trade was respect. When they get respect they exchange it for information, knowledge, resources and goodwill. Failure to give respect can be met with revenge strategies in the form of an embargo of trade.

Although many sources call for clear policies and procedures so that roles on the team are clear, there are also more subtle rules of the game that will never appear in a manual. One resident stated it like this: "Your name can be ruined or made on one encounter—you have to be very careful, because if you create one enemy you can end up having a tough time with a lot of people and if they love you, then they love you for all the time you are there" (Lingaard et al 2004).

Tips for improving collegial relationships

- Cultivate personal attributes such as the ability to accept differences, take risks, function independently, articulate roles, and tolerate reviews and challenges of your ideas.
- Take some time to form relationships with your colleagues.
- Treat others with integrity, honesty and respect.
- Take the lead in fostering the idea that we are all in this together.
- Master the principles of interprofessional collegiality.

Summary

Health care has rapidly evolved and is now delivered by teams of professionals. Physicians for whom this is a shift in their accustomed practise style will benefit from reflecting on the role they have with a team of fellow health practitioners. In such settings, it is ineffective, disruptive, and potentially dangerous to view one's practice as unique and outside of the function of the team. Thus, the development of collegial relationships with team members not only improves care to patients, but also improves the health and satisfaction of all members of the team, including physicians.

Case resolution

After the resident speaks to the fellow about the situation, the fellow offers to speak to the nurse on her behalf. The resident wanted to deal with this herself so waited until she and the nurse were alone and raised the issue with the nurse. The resident told the nurse she was surprised and angry when her request was ignored and was concerned that the patient could have suffered if the fellow had not been available. The nurse could not really explain her behaviour but did say she saw the resident as "one of them" and "not as a physician to take charge in an emergency." She did admit that the resident's approach to the problem was correct and that she was sorry for her behaviour.

The resident begins to question her friendliness with the nursing staff and wondered if she needed to set herself apart from them but decided that she would keep talking about this issue with other colleagues and nurses.

Key references

Lingaard L, Espin S, Evans C, Hawryluck L. 2004. The rules of the game: interprofessional collaboration on the intensive care unit team. *Critical Care*. 8: R403–8.

Spagnoletti CL and RM Arnold. 2007. R-E-S-P-E-C-T: even more difficult to teach than to define. *Journal of General Internal Medicine*. 22 (5): 707–9.

Introduction: Physician health and the doctor–patient relationship

Leslie Flynn, MD MMus CCFP FRCPC

The physician–patient relationship is central to the practise of modern medicine. The hierarchical model of care that was accepted in the past is outmoded in today's patient-centred health care system. The fundamental principles of the Canadian Medical Association's Code of Ethics emphasize that the physician is to "[f]irst consider the well-being of the patient" and to "[p]ractice the profession of medicine in a manner that treats the patient with dignity and as a person worthy of respect." The fulfilment of these principles is essential for the delivery of high-quality medical care.

Patients are active participants in their care; they value autonomy, ready access to information, and participation in decision-making. It is important also to appreciate that the contemporary physician–patient relationship is fiduciary in nature; it is based on the expectation of trustworthiness, the requirement that the interaction will occur under conditions of confidentiality and privacy, and the recognition that an unequal power relationship exists. The following observations take each of these features in turn.

Trust. The physician is responsible for creating an environment of mutual respect and trust. By creating a safe environment and earning trust, physicians will enjoy a collaborative and productive relationship with patients. Reviewing key tenets of informed consent, appropriately sharing information and decisions, and inviting patients to share their perspectives and beliefs will promote quality care.

Privacy. Confidentiality and privacy are critical to the practice of medicine. Through policies that respect the scope and limits of confidentiality and privacy, physicians facilitate the development of a healthy relationship with their patients.

Power. The power differential between physician and patient is always weighted in the physician's favour. Patients are vulnerable by virtue of having a health concern, which is often coupled with fear or anxiety. Physicians have extensive knowledge, the authority to diagnose and treat, and the responsibility to make difficult recommendations and interventions. By being mindful of this power differential and doing all that is reasonable to facilitate patient autonomy, physicians promote a healthy relationship with their patients.

Physicians treating physicians

The doctor whose patient is a physician faces particular challenges. This is a dual relationship—the treating physician will naturally relate to the patient as a peer, as well as in the role of doctor. The patient may be a close colleague, such as a clinician in the department. They may be a distant acquaintance, but one who sits on the same board meetings or on the same hospital medical advisory committee. The patient may be a physician of renown, well recognized as an expert clinician with exemplary diagnostic skill.

These possibilities can threaten the treating physician's ability to be objective. In a typical clinical situation the doctor is assured that they have a superior knowledge base to rely on when interacting with the patient. To feel otherwise can be disconcerting. The doctor treating another doctor may wonder: "Do I know enough to treat this patient?" An expectation that the patient has extensive knowledge, paired with the treating physician's self-doubt, can lead to inadequate care in the form of a poor, superficial history, an abbreviated physical exam and a lack of attention to provide comprehensive patient education.

Further, this dual relationship can induce an unspoken expectation that special treatment will be provided. Certainly, professional courtesy has existed within medicine since the time of Hippocrates. This phrase refers to the provision of care to physician colleagues before other patients and/or, in jurisdictions other than Canada, at a reduced rate. Although not an ethical requirement, this practise was established as a means of assisting those within the profession to access care and sustain their practice. Professional courtesy does not include treatment that changes the nature and manner in which the care is provided. This includes for example changes such as providing appointments outside of regular clinic hours or making home visits when not warranted. These are the changes in the nature or manner in which care is typically provided.

The treating physician in this scenario must ensure that they provide the same high standard of care to the physician patient that any other patient would receive. This means not letting one's guard down by, for example, allowing physician patients to write their own prescriptions, change the dose of their medications without consultation, or arrange for their own investigations. In addition, the treating physician should not assume that the doctor patient is aware of the typical medical management of their condition and thus be less than diligent in obtaining informed consent.

These types of lapses are boundary violations. Although it is appropriate to be respectful of one's colleague and acknowledge their professional status, it is essential to adhere to one's usual patterns of practice. A loss of objectivity can threaten the care provided; challenging situations such as communicating bad news, addressing issues of substance use and abuse, or identifying concerns regarding compliance with treatment can become too difficult to negotiate.

Being a physician to physicians requires the capacity to monitor one's own emotional reactions. This awareness will help the treating physician manage this relationship in a responsible and professional manner. In addition, maintaining an open approach to discussing roles and expectations will be beneficial for both parties. Finally, as with all patients, it is important, with the patient's consent, to involve the patient's spouse or partner in treatment planning. Spouses who are not physicians already feel isolated when their physician partner is ill, given their lack of medical knowledge. Involving them early on in the process of management can help them in their supportive role.

Physicians being patients

Moving from a position of authority (practising physician) to a position that feels exposed and vulnerable (physician patient) can be uncomfortable; physicians who find themselves in this position may fear a loss of autonomy and control and worry about the potential for a breach of privacy. These fears can lead physicians to delay seeking care, or to minimize symptoms or aspects of their medical history. This jeopardizes the treating physician's ability to provide appropriate care and may, in turn, put the physician patient's health at risk.

Complete confidentiality is important for any patient. For physicians, there is a particular need to be guaranteed that their medical record will be kept confidential. This is particularly the case in relation to problems that are stigmatized, such as mental illness, substance misuse or blood-borne disease (e.g., HIV). Issues that may jeopardize the patient's competence to practise are especially delicate. The patient must have a physician who can be honest and forthright in a sensitive, empathic and caring fashion. The physician must be careful that their own personal beliefs and perspectives do not interfere with effective care.

Physicians are sensitive to the workload of their colleagues. They may not wish to impose upon a colleague or to add to the stresses present in an overburdened health care system. This viewpoint can lead physicians to negate their own need for health care, even for periodic monitoring. It is essential that all medical students, residents and practising physicians be encouraged to establish a relationship with a family physician and make regular health care one of their priorities. This connection to a family physician can provide a valuable support in dealing with the stresses of a medical career and facilitate access to health care when needed.

Summary

Being a physician in need of care, or being a physician who is asked to provide care to another physician, can be difficult scenarios for those involved. It is clear that the treating physician must provide patient-centred care. Physicians must be caring, listen carefully and communicate clearly, facilitate collaboration and provide a high standard of timely care. The patient desires expert care in an environment of trust. Confidentiality is central to the practice of medicine and must be maintained. Physicians need health promotion and disease prevention services. They also become ill and will require care. In such situations, both doctor and patient must demonstrate and expect mutual respect.

Key references

Bleiberg E. 2003. Treating professionals in crisis: a framework focused on promoting mentalizing. *Bulletin of the Menninger Clinic.* 67 (3): 212–6.

Canadian Medical Association. 2004. *Code of Ethics.*[policy]. Ottawa: The CMA.

Gabbard GO and C Nadelson. 1995. Professional boundaries in the physician–patient relationship. *Journal of the American Medical Association.* 273 (18): 1445–9. Published erratum appears in: *JAMA.* 1995; 274 (17): 1346.

A. Coping with an adverse event, complaint or litigation

Canadian Medical Protective Association

Objectives

This chapter will

- discuss the effects of medical errors, complaints and litigation on physicians in training and throughout their career in medicine, and
- present an approach to dealing with errors and complaints in medicine.

Case

During a busy day a young physician is served with a statement of claim. The legal claim is made by the family of a 59-year-old woman, a patient the physician had seen and discharged, who died of a myocardial infarct later the same day.

The physician scans the document quickly but has to get back to work. The physician has difficulty completing the shift and experiences feelings of insecurity bordering on panic. Although the physician believes his family will be supportive, the physician is ashamed to tell them about the legal action and the mistakes the physician presumes to have made in the case.

Introduction

Every physician in Canada is likely to be affected by a medico-legal issue at some point over the course of their career. Approximately two per cent of physicians are named in a legal action each year. Far more are involved in a wide variety of other medico-legal difficulties. Patients or other parties may complain about a physician to a regulatory authority (college), hospital or privacy commissioner or to the Human Rights Commission. Physicians may be referred for college disciplinary hearings or have their practice reviewed. Hospital disputes and conflicts can involve doctors. On occasion, criminal accusations are lodged against a physician.

Medico-legal difficulties are stressful for physicians for several reasons. In some cases, the problem arises from a clinical outcome that is unexpected and even disastrous to the patient. It is normal for a doctor to feel distressed when a patient dies unexpectedly or suffers a serious complication. Physicians experience empathy and sorrow for the patient and family when a tragic clinical outcome occurs. Sometimes sorrow becomes mixed with guilt. Doctors may beat up on themselves and wonder, in hindsight, whether they should have done something differently to avert the poor outcome. They may be tormented by doubts and second thoughts, even if their management of the case, viewed prospectively, had appeared reasonable at the time.

Physicians invest inordinate amounts of time and energy in their work, and their self-image is often centred on their status as a physician. Legal allegations and patient complaints frequently depict doctors as callous, negligent or incompetent; physicians may feel this is a direct assault on their essence as a person. In the face of an adverse event, complaint or legal action, physicians often harbour visions of disastrous personal consequences, such as the loss of reputation, desertion by patients, suspension of hospital privileges or revocation of their medical licence. They may also dread the possibility of media coverage of the clinical event, their trial, or college hearing.

Physicians' reactions to medico-legal difficulties

Internal emotions

- sorrow
- guilt
- loss of self-esteem
- shame
- fear

External pressures

- social isolation from friends and family
- lack of knowledge of legal/regulatory process
- perceived or real lack of hospital/collegial support
- potential for media exposure

Physicians are also susceptible to feelings of isolation during difficult moments in their career. Heavy workloads can make it hard to maintain a social network of friends and colleagues with whom they can commiserate and share experiences. They may also feel shame or embarrassment about presumed medical errors. Many strive for perfection; viewing an adverse event as a failure, they may be inclined to keep the matter from their colleagues.

Maintaining perspective

Although it is impossible to erase a physician's sadness and regret associated with a poor patient outcome, feelings of guilt, inadequacy or fear can be greatly attenuated by keeping the matter in perspective. Physicians may be consoled by the following facts and observations.

A poor patient outcome, even if unexpected, does not signify that a medical error has occurred. A delayed or missed diagnosis or a surgical complication does not equate with negligence. In law, a doctor is not expected to be perfect. Canadian courts have determined that the clinical standard of care by which a claim is judged is not one of perfection, but rather one that might reasonably be expected from a normal, prudent health care provider of similar training and experience in similar circumstances.

Sometimes, however, physicians involved in a medico-legal issue have made a mistake, such as diagnostic, management or technical error, or failure to notice or act on a laboratory or imaging result.

Although physicians strive for excellence, it is helpful to accept the fact of every clinician's fallibility. Doctors are human, and no one is perfect. In spite of a deep commitment to patient care and the best intentions, poor outcomes may, unfortunately, be related to health care delivery itself.

Doctors often work in suboptimal conditions; they may be overloaded with work and may suffer from fatigue or sleep deprivation. A physician may be loath to use fatigue as an excuse for a poor outcome, but the reality is that fatigue and other system and organizational issues often contribute to the occurrence of adverse events.

All colleagues and most patients are aware that any physician, even the most competent and knowledgeable among them, may encounter a medico-legal difficulty at one time or another. It is unusual for patients to leave a physician's practice because of another patient's complaint or legal action. Colleagues, patients, other health professionals, family and friends are appreciative of a physician who is caring, conscientious and committed to his or her work. Their appreciation and support of the physician are rarely affected by a medico-legal difficulty.

Physicians' worries about the effect of a lawsuit or patient complaint on their career are often exaggerated. However, even when the medico-legal problem is reported in the media, in most cases it is quickly forgotten by all but the parties involved.

There is, of course, no magic remedy for the regret and sadness experienced by physicians about poor patient outcomes; these are burdens that all physicians carry, and are never forgotten.

Managing the stress

Physicians should not be ashamed to seek help when facing a medico-legal difficulty. Canadian Medical Protective Association (CMPA) members who receive a statement of claim or college complaint should call the Association right away. Medical officers at the CMPA are sensitive to the stresses engendered by an adverse event and medico-legal difficulties, and are pleased to listen to and support members suffering from uncertainty and worry. Medical officers and/or CMPA legal counsel will explain the legal process to the member. Knowing what to expect allows the doctor to prepare and feel more in control, which usually diminishes anxiety. The stages of a legal action in Canada and strategies for coping with the stress involved are also described on the CMPA website (www.cmpa-acpm.ca/cmpapd04/docs/publications/com_education-e.cfm - click on "Legal proceedings").

Nor should physicians feel inhibited from consulting their own family physician, who will usually understand and empathize with the feelings of a physician patient grappling with a medico-legal problem. Friends, colleagues and family are also usually understanding and supportive. However, the specifics of the case should be discussed only with the CMPA medical officer, or with the CMPA lawyer if the matter has been referred to counsel, so as to maintain legal privilege.

Provincial and university- or community-based physician health programs are available to provide support and assistance to physicians going through difficult moments. Contact information is available in Chapter 12-B of this guide.

Practical considerations

Most physicians do cope reasonably well with adverse events and medico-legal issues. Many come to realize that a medico-legal difficulty is not the cataclysmic event they may have imagined. A medico-legal difficulty may induce a physician to appraise their practice and lifestyle and to implement constructive changes. Doctors should endeavour to achieve a satisfying work–life balance, and if a phase of practice becomes particularly stressful they may wish to modify their practice to allow for more time to invest in and take care of themselves. They should not self-medicate or use substances or alcohol to alleviate stress. It can also be helpful to engage the services of a coach, counsellor or therapist to help them approach and process the complexity of issues being faced.

Positive practice changes can enhance patient safety, but physicians should also avoid the urge to practise overly defensive medicine with excessive and clinically unwarranted investigations. Above all, physicians should strive to do their best, to be thorough and conscientious, and to realize that perfection is unattainable.

Case resolution

The physician's spouse is also a family physician and is unwavering in their support during the legal process. Kind words from colleagues and patients helped to restore the physician's confidence in themselves and the system. The physician institutes some changes in their approach to certain patient complaints and regains a sense of work satisfaction.

Key reference

Delbanco T and SK Bell. 2007. Guilty, afraid, and alone—Struggling with medical error. *New England Journal of Medicine.* 357 (17): 1682–3.

B. Coping when values collide

Merril Pauls, MD MHSc CCFP(EM)

Objectives

This chapter will

- describe the difference between personal and professional values,
- outline the professional and legal standards that frame the options physicians have in dealing with value conflicts with a patient, and
- present ways to resolve such differences while optimizing patient care.

> **Case**
>
> A senior obstetrics and gynecology resident agrees to do an optional rotation at a fertility clinic. A lesbian couple approaches the clinic requesting in vitro fertilization using donor sperm. According to the resident's religious beliefs, homosexuality is wrong and children should have both a mother and a father. The resident is not willing to participate in the provision of this care.

Introduction

We all have beliefs that shape our view of the world and influence our actions. Because these views differ from person to person, they can give rise to conflict. This is particularly problematic in the context of a physician–patient relationship. Physicians and patients enter into this relationship with the understanding that the needs of the patient will take precedence. But does this mean the physician should leave his or her values at the door? Although physicians should be able to practise in a manner consistent with their personal beliefs, they must still meet the standards and expectations of their profession. In the event of a conflict of values it is crucial that physicians understand their own beliefs, explore the expectations of their patients, and familiarize themselves with relevant professional standards.

The conscientious objection debate

In today's pluralistic society there are a number of legally available and medically acceptable treatments that contravene the moral code or religious beliefs of particular physicians. Can a physician refuse to participate in these treatments on the basis of a conscientious objection? Examples include providing or referring a patient for a therapeutic abortion, prescribing post-coital contraception, and providing in vitro fertilization services to certain patients. The appropriate way for a physician to manage these situations is controversial and currently under debate. The issue of therapeutic abortion has been most widely discussed and explored in this regard.

Those who oppose a physician's right to conscientious objection argue that physicians have been trained by society and have a fiduciary duty to their patients. They express the concern that if physicians were allowed to "opt out," it would inevitably happen that some patients would not be able to find a physician in their area who is willing to provide a given service, thus preventing them from accessing legitimate treatments.

Others have argued that even if physicians are allowed to refuse to participate in a procedure on moral or religious grounds they must disclose their position and refer the patient to a provider who is willing to provide the procedure.

On the other side of the debate are those who say that the moral and religious beliefs that underpin most conscientious objections are shared by a large segment of the population. Physicians with certain beliefs should not be excluded from the practice of medicine. They argue that physicians are more than technicians; they are moral agents whose beliefs and values should receive some consideration. Many physicians have argued that the Human Rights Code should protect the rights of patients, but also protect the right of physicians not to be discriminated against for their beliefs.

The Canadian Medical Association's policy on induced abortion states that a physician should be allowed to both agree to provide, and to refuse to participate in, induced abortion without being discriminated against. It also says that physicians whose beliefs prevent them from recommending or providing an abortion should inform the patient of this, so that she can consult another physician if she chooses. It does not state that the physician must refer the patient to another physician or assist her in finding another physician—a subject that has generated much debate (Rodgers and Downie 2006). More recently, the College of Physicians and Surgeons of Ontario (CPSO) has developed a policy on Physicians and the Ontario Human Rights Code. They suggest that physicians who decline to provide a medical service on the basis of gender, sexual orientation or a number of other prohibited grounds (identified in the Human Rights Code and the Canadian Charter of Rights and Freedoms) will be seen as contravening the Ontario code. The fact that their refusal is based in moral or religious beliefs would not constitute a defence. This CPSO policy also states the professional expectations for Ontario physicians:

> "communicate clearly and promptly with patients about treatments one is unwilling to provide; do not withhold information from patients about treatments that conflict with one's personal beliefs; do not express personal judgments about a patient's lifestyle or choices; advise patients that they may see another physician if they choose; and help them make arrangements to do so."

Some elements are generally agreed upon with regard to conscientious objection in medicine, and physicians should use these to guide their decision-making:

- You must provide treatment to a patient requiring urgent or emergent care, even if the situation has arisen from a treatment you would object to (e.g., a woman who is bleeding after a therapeutic abortion).
- You must disclose to patients that you are not prepared to participate in certain procedures should they become relevant to the patient's clinical situation. This should occur as early as possible and should be done in a non-judgmental way.
- You must inform the patient that there are different views regarding these matters in the medical community and that they may see another physician if they choose.
- If the treatment or procedure is time-sensitive (e.g., it loses effectiveness or options becomes more limited with the passage of time) this should be explained to the patient.
- Physicians who work in an institution or in a setting where the treatment or procedure would normally be available should disclose their concerns to their employer or clinical chief and negotiate an appropriate approach before seeing patients.
- Medical students or residents should discuss their concerns with the institution and their clinical chief before starting their rotation. Most institutions have policies in this regard.

The most contentious issues are whether a physician must assist the patient in accessing the treatment (e.g., refer the patient to another physician who will provide the treatment) and whether conscientious objection should be allowed in those situations where there is no other way for a patient to access a treatment (e.g., if all the physicians in a community refuse to perform abortions). Some physicians believe that even generating a referral makes them complicit in the provision of a treatment or procedure that they believe to be wrong, and point to the CMA *Code of Ethics* to suggest they do not have a responsibility to do so. However, some provincial colleges may consider this to fall below the standard of care should a complaint arise.

Summary

Although a patient's choices should not be limited by a physician's moral or religious beliefs, it is unrealistic to suggest that an individual physician should participate in a procedure to which he or she objects when no willing physician is available. It also seems unlikely that an individual physician would face sanction in this situation, even though it is an unacceptable situation for the patient. Often an institution or region will have to provide the resources needed to connect the patient to the procedure in a timely manner (e.g., send a patient to another community to obtain an abortion).

Some additional suggestions may lead to a more satisfactory resolution of these situations for physicians and their patients. If you are contemplating a conscientious objection, you should understand and explore the scientific and moral basis for it. This will help you clarify when and where you should take a stand.

Be as proactive as possible. Let your employer/institution and colleagues know your intent. Develop a plan to address different ways in which the issue may arise. Let your patients know as soon as is feasible.

Although it is not acceptable to judge a patient's choices, or attempt to convert them to your beliefs, it is acceptable to express concern for the patient and to offer to continue to provide care for them in other areas.

Case resolution

In this case, although the resident has deeply held religious convictions, the basis for denying the service (sexual orientation) is clearly identified in the Human Rights Code as a prohibited ground for doing so. The resident immediately goes to their supervisor and explains that they feel they cannot participate in the requested procedure. The supervisor takes over the case and provides the service the couple is seeking. After discussion with the program director it is decided that the resident should not complete the elective, and decides not to include IVF in their practice. The resident is still able to complete residency, qualifies as an obstetrician and gynecologist, and now ensures that their patients know the limits of their practice.

Key references

Canadian Medical Association. *Induced Abortion* [policy]. Last retrieved from CMA's website: June 25, 2009: policybase.cma.ca/dbtw-wpd/PolicyPDF/PD88-06.pdf.

College of Physicians and Surgeons of Ontario. 2008. *Physicians and the Ontario Human Rights Code* [policy #5-08]. Last retrieved June 25, 2009, from CPSO's website: www.cpso.on.ca/uploadedFiles/downloads/cpsodocuments/policies/policies/human_rights.pdf.

Rodgers S and J Downie. 2006. Abortion: ensuring access [editorial]. *Canadian Medical Association Journal.* 175 (1): 9.

C. Coping with challenging patient behaviour

Derek Puddester, MD MEd FRCPC

Objectives

This chapter will

- describe challenging patient behaviours, and
- summarize methods of preventing or managing these behaviours.

Case

A second-year resident attends to a patient who, in spite of appropriate and excellent care, develops significant medical complications. When the resident shares this news with the patient and his family, the resident is verbally abused and begins to fear for their own safety. For the next few weeks, conversations with the patient and family are difficult, and the hurtful nature of the engagement worsens. Family members begin to discuss information about the resident found online and start to make threatening remarks about the resident's family. The resident feels unsafe and is uncertain about how best to proceed.

Introduction

Taking the role of patient can be an uncomfortable situation for many people. When we do find ourselves in this role, our emotions may range from simple irritation to frank terror. Few of us like to be confronted by our vulnerabilities and, even less, by our mortality. It is natural not to want anything to stand in the way of life. Meanwhile, physicians are often the bearers of bad news. Although a physician's role is to help the patient, the very fact that they are needed is in almost every circumstance unwelcome.

Other factors contribute to the inherent tensions of the physician–patient relationship. For example, patients bring beliefs and expectations to the encounter that may not be consonant with the physician's expertise. At times patients may feel that their perspective is being dismissed. And finally, along with their physicians, patients are faced with the stresses of accessing care within a health care system that is complex and strained.

These stressors can cause difficulties in communication and collaboration to arise. This chapter will outline some of the critical aspects of patient–physician conflict and present strategies to reduce risk.

Verbal aggression

Aggression can be triggered by many emotions, perhaps the most common of which is fear. If a patient or family member becomes verbally aggressive, acknowledge their feelings gently but clearly. Ask what they would find helpful at that moment. At the same time, ask them to help you by remaining calm. In other cases, verbal aggression may be a presenting sign of an underlying pathology and can be useful in differential diagnosis. In such cases, do everything possible to offer appropriate interventions.

If your best efforts are not successful, consider offering an apology (e.g., "I am sorry that I haven't been able to resolve this issue for you") and alert your supervisor. In some situations, the patient or family member might respond only to someone they perceive to have more authority. In such cases, do not take the situation personally. The issues at play are theirs, not yours. Return to observe how your supervisor manages the situation and see if you can re-engage in a collaborative relationship with the patient or family member.

Key strategies to ensure physical safety

- Request that your program offer training in non-violent crisis intervention.
- Ensure that others know where you are at all times.
- Know the situation. Ask colleagues for an update, and read the chart before seeing the patient.
- Learn how to read the signs of imminent aggression.
- Acknowledge the person's distress and ask what you can do to help.
- Be aware of all exits from an interview or assessment area.
- If you perceive danger, terminate the interview and exit. Immediately seek help, including from security staff or police as needed.
- If you are seeing a violent or aggressive patient be aware of the standard protocol for intervention, whether verbal, chemical or physical.

Threats

Patients or family members sometimes feel wronged or acutely frustrated at not getting what they want. This may provoke them to make physical threats or to challenge your professional status by threatening to resort to formal complaint or legal action. Offer to listen to the concerns of the patient or family member again. Perhaps you've missed something and by acknowledging that you can minimize the threat. Encourage the person to put his or her concerns and desired outcomes in writing. Consider inviting a third party such as your chief resident or supervisor to help. Finally, respect any request to make a complaint by directing the person to the appropriate channels and indicating that feedback is welcome.

Intimidation

It is important to have insight into your own responses to being bullied. Some people are uncomfortable with conflict and to avoid confrontation become submissive. In a patient care situation, this can be unprofessional (e.g., if a patient demands unnecessary interventions). Others respond to bullying with a strong reaction that may be experienced by the patient as abusive.

In general, remaining neutral is best. Clearly explain that you want to work collaboratively with the patient, and offer the best care possible. Emphasize what you are, or are not, willing to do and why. If appropriate, indicate that you can arrange for the patient to be seen by another physician if he or she prefers. If care is ongoing, consider asking your supervisor or another member of the team to join you when you see the patient. Consistently ask the patient to clarify their expectations and do what is reasonable to meet them. Remind the patient of what you cannot do and why. Document your observations and interventions and ensure that your supervisor is aware of the situation.

Privacy issues

All of us leave a digital imprint wherever we go, and in some cases (e.g., physician rating sites) imprints are created about us. It is important to be aware of your imprint and the information it contains. If highly personal information about you or your loved ones is readily available on the web, it can be found by others and used maliciously. Such situations are stressful and potentially harmful.

Maximize your privacy by being cautious about the sort of personal information you put on the web, including social networking sites (e.g., Facebook, MySpace, Twitter). Set your privacy settings as high as possible and restrict access to known friends or family members. Request that they do not post information about you or your loved ones without explicit permission. From time to time, do a web search on your name. It is not uncommon for physicians to be surprised at the volume of personal and professional information that can easily be collected online. Depending on the site, you may be able to request that information be removed or modified; however, this is not always possible, especially if you have agreed to the terms of use for a particular site.

Finally, what might have been fun to post when you were an undergraduate or medical student can be unhelpful as you seek academic appointments or fellowships. Increasingly, training institutions and employers search social networking sites as part of routine screening. At the end of the day, you are in control of what you post and share. What you cannot control is how others respond to what they find.

Physical violence

All physicians require training in the assessment and management of violent behaviour. If this is not offered as part of your residency training program, ask your program director to arrange for a skills-oriented workshop. A widely recognized certification program offered by the Crisis Prevention Institute (www.crisisprevention.com) teaches practical skills to assess and manage violence in a multitude of settings.

In general, the least experienced members of the team are the most at risk of being injured. Do not intervene in a situation unless you have been appropriately trained. A violent patient or family member represents a serious emergency; alert the rest of the team, including your supervisor, and request their immediate intervention. Finally, be mindful that any medical students you may be supervising are at particular risk of harm.

Critical incident debriefing

Critical incidents can have a profound impact on everyone involved. Critical incident debriefing is a voluntary process that allows individuals to discuss an incident from a personal or professional perspective. Facilitated by trained experts, such sessions are not about assigning blame or investigating errors. Rather, they allow for safe discussion of the incident and normalization of the complex emotions they provoke. If you are not included in a debriefing session that is relevant to you and would like to have access to this service, make your wishes known. Not processing the feelings associated with a critical incident can be harmful to you and your practice. Seek support and mentorship early and quickly. You'll be glad you did.

Case resolution

The resident eventually reports the strained nature of the relationship to their supervisor, who immediately arranges for a meeting between the patient, his family and the medical team. With the patient's permission, the hospital's Patient Representative is invited to attend. The meeting is difficult, but it reveals that the family had misunderstood a critical component of the care offered to the patient and had mistakenly blamed the resident for the outcome. Once clarified, the family offered an apology to the team and acknowledged regret about their behaviour. The rapport between the resident and the family continued to be guarded but was much more respectful. The resident also took an opportunity to review and modify their web presence and noted surprise at the volume of personal information found online.

Key references

Haas LJ, Leiser JP, Magill MK, Sanyer ON. 2005. Management of the difficult patient. *American Family Physician.* 72: 2063–8.

Hawken SJ. 2005. Strategies for dealing with the challenging patient. *New Zealand Family Physician.* 32 (4): 266–9.

D. Boundary issues

Michael Paré, MD MEd

Objectives

This chapter will

- define boundary, boundary crossing and boundary violation,
- discuss the importance of boundaries in physician–patient relationships, and
- examine how the maintenance of healthy boundaries can promote physician sustainability and the quality of care.

Case

A third-year family practice resident is following a 15-year-old female patient for suspected depression and bulimia. During a follow-up appointment she expresses disappointment and frustration with her body, noting "I'm as flat as the Sahara desert." The resident gives supportive feedback that she has a normal physical appearance, seems to be progressing normally through puberty, and "has nice, well-developed breasts for a girl of her age." The girl is visibly upset by this comment and complains to her parents, who report the resident to the college.

Introduction

From the time of the Hippocratic oath, maintaining boundaries was established as an important core of professional practice. This is made clear in the Oath which requires that the physician will conduct himself or herself "In purity and holiness," will treat the sick, "will keep them from harm and injustice," and will "come for the benefit of the sick, remaining free of all intentional injustice, of all mischief and in particular of sexual relations with both female and male persons."

Boundaries clarify the necessary distance between the doctor and the patient. Keeping healthy boundaries is often automatic and usually easy but can at times be difficult for both patient and physician. It is important for the profession to have detailed guidelines and limits for appropriate boundary behaviour and equally important to allow the for the doctor-patient relationship to be reasonably flexible—in keeping with any genuine and dynamic relationship.

What are boundaries?

1. Boundaries elucidate the roles and expectations involved in the physician–patient relationship.
2. Boundaries clarify the pertinent therapeutic distance between physician and patient.
3. Boundaries thus define the limits of the therapeutic relationship.

Occasionally, physicians are required to negotiate difficult and sensitive boundaries. At times this is described as "dancing along the boundary." This flexibility needs to be done in a reflective and thoughtful manner in order to ensure that boundaries are maintained.

Boundary crossings and boundary violations

Boundary issues encompass both boundary crossings and boundary violations. The occurrence of either should be the cause of some potential concern.

Boundary Crossing: A boundary can be crossed without being violated. Many boundary crossings are benign. In fact, it is entirely possible that a boundary may be consciously crossed with the intention and actuality of assisting the treatment in some way. In fact, boundary crossings may, at times, indicate an exceptional, innovative and/or an intuitive departure from the common treatment protocol. However, at other times, boundary crossings may occur because of carelessness or a lack of thought.

Boundary Violation: A boundary violation is far more serious than a boundary crossing. Boundary violations harm the patient in some way. By definition, a boundary crossing becomes a boundary violation when the result is harm to the patient.

Boundaries, once established, ought not to be readily crossed. However, crossings do occur and often do not do harm to either the practitioner or the patient. Should harm come from a boundary crossing, the action is then defined as a boundary violation.

The determination of harm is generally determined by acceptable practice as defined by the patient and the public. For example, sexual behaviour with a patient is widely acknowledged as harmful. Gently encouraging a patient to quit smoking and triggering an angry and defensive reaction, is widely acknowledged not to be harmful.

Boundary crossings may, at times, simply be communication blunders. At other times, they indicate an innovative or an intuitive departure from the common treatment protocol. What may cross a boundary in one relationship may be perfectly acceptable in another. Boundaries are often very subjective and very much depend on the context. For example, casually addressing each other using first names could be fine in many relationships (e.g., between medical colleagues), and unacceptable in others (e.g., an elderly, very conservative female patient who insists on being addressed as: Mrs. Gertrude Green, rather than simply as "Gertrude", or worse yet: "Gertie").

Therapeutic frame

Boundaries between doctor and patient are particularly important since they define the therapeutic frame. The development of a therapeutic frame is an important way that the concept of boundaries is used in a clinical setting. What is within this frame is effective and ethical treatment; what is outside this frame is ineffective and/or unethical intervention. The idea here is that treatment must take place within a structural and conceptual space defined by certain parameters.

Other words that could be used to convey this are: "the rules" and "the norms" of the therapeutic encounter, which help define a therapeutic milieu that is beneficial to the development of a therapeutic experience. These are conceived as necessary, yet certainly not sufficient conditions, for the provision of successful, high-quality treatment. Note also that in crossing the line of effective treatment, the physician may enter a "gray zone" (or more optimistically a "pastel zone") that is somewhat indeterminate in terms of either positive or negative effects on the treatment. Entering this gray or pastel zone may, at times, be helpful, yet it is always risky and certainly could be detrimental. Although most boundary transgressions are conceptualized as being "over" the boundary (the doctor is intrusive or the abusive), it is important to realize that sometimes the doctor is "under-involved" (the doctor is cold or rejecting) with their patient.

Guthiel and Gabbard's article, *The concept of boundaries in clinical practice: Theoretical and risk-management dimensions*, is an excellent overview of boundary issues. The article articulates well what clinical boundaries are and the need to respect them. There are pertinent boundaries for the many various facets of the doctor patient relationship. These boundary facets include, but are not limited to

- social role,
- time,
- place and space,
- money,
- gifts and services,
- clothing,
- language,
- self-disclosure, and
- physical contact.

Since self-disclosure is such an important boundary and since the case included an unwise self-disclosure it is worthwhile to briefly cover this topic.

Physician self-disclosure

Most physicians would agree that sharing some personal details with a patient is necessary and even helpful. However, revealing personal information may lead to disclosing increasingly intimate and potentially sensitive information. It is this practise that has the probability of turning from a boundary crossing to a boundary violation.

Four useful practical principles of physician self-disclosure have been suggested. These principles are as follows:

1. Physicians should remember that it is for the patients' needs that they reveal themselves; therefore, physicians should reveal themselves judiciously.
2. When physicians self-disclose they should always consider the current stage the relationship is in (later in the doctor-patient relationship somewhat more self-disclosure is usually okay).
3. Physicians should not disclose those things that are a source of emotional conflict within themselves.
4. Physicians should think about how their self-disclosure would sound to other people.

Summary

Maintaining good boundaries is central to quality care. By setting, and then following reasonably clear and appropriate boundaries, physicians make their life easier and simpler, and increase their sense of joy in the practice of medicine.

Case resolution

The resident is an outstanding resident with no history of boundary issues. The resident agrees that this particular incident was a boundary crossing, and if not well managed could be perceived as a boundary violation. The resident acknowledges that the wording of the comment was awkward, inappropriate and clearly it was not helpful to the patient. In reviewing the principles of physician self-disclosure, the resident realizes that what was disclosed did not sound appropriate to either the patient or her parents. The resident offers to meet with the family in the presence of a supervisor to apologize and explain this error. The meeting is tense but helpful; the family express that the comments were seen as inappropriate and harmful but also acknowledge that it was intended to support the patient and normalize her self-image. The resident acknowledges that the words were hurtful and demonstrates how to handle a similar situation differently. The complaint is dropped, the resident is more mindful of their use of language in discussing sensitive subjects, and the patient remains in the resident's care.

Key references

Gutheil TG and GO Gabbard. 1993. The concept of boundaries in clinical practice: Theoretical and risk-management dimensions. *American Journal of Psychiatry*. 150: 188–96.

Paré M. 2001. Boundaries in primary care medicine. *Patient Care Canada*. 12 (10): 76–112.

Introduction: The physician life-cycle

Jordan Cohen, MD FRCPC

The life-cycle of a physician is a complex process of development. At a basic level, medical education must occur in a specific sequence for the learner to move successfully from one level to the next. At the same time, the learning and acquisition of experience through which students become residents and then practising physicians is multi-layered. The Royal College CanMEDS Framework endeavours to ensure that all physicians develop basic core competencies in all of their Roles (Medical Expert, Communicator, Collaborator, Health Advocate, Manager, Scholar, and Professional), but each individual, depending on the degree to which he or she chooses to emphasize each of these Roles within their career, becomes a unique physician.

The major transitions that occur in the education of a physician are the move from medical school training to residency, from residency to practice, and from active practice to eventual retirement. Depending on the type of practice environment that they have chosen, a physician may make different stops along the way. For example, a physician who has chosen to establish her own practice and focus on clinical aspects of medicine will not encounter some of the expectations and pressures of a full-time faculty member, who is expected to participate in academia and to contribute to scholarly research. Depending on a physician's choice of career and personal interests, they will diversify to varying degrees in clinical work, teaching, administration and research.

Figure 3. The physician's life-cycle

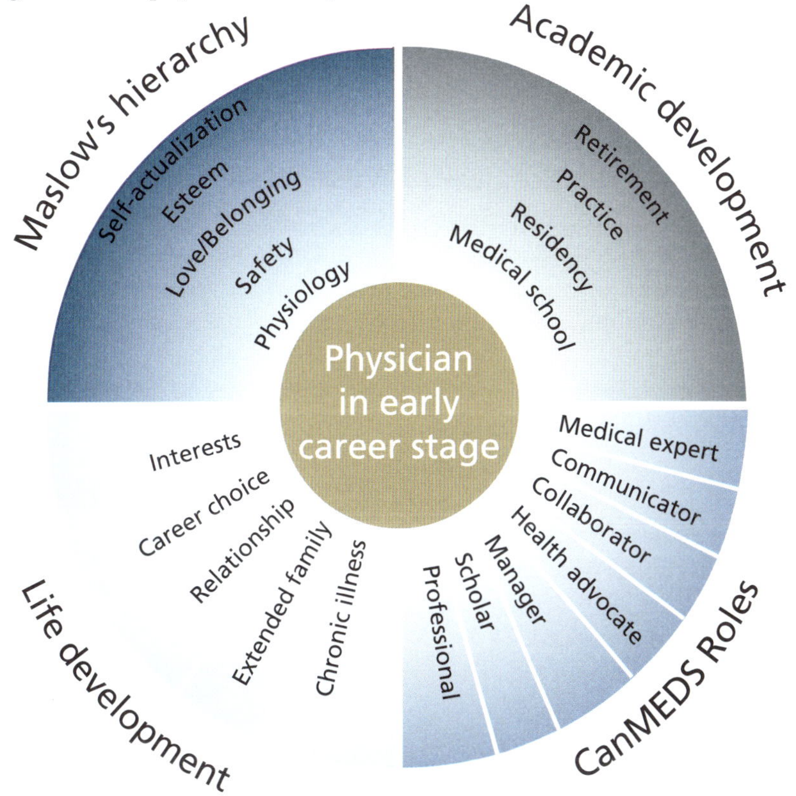

A further layer of growth involves the personal aspect of one's life, such as intimate relationships, plans to have a family, health issues and the needs of family members.

Self-reflection on the personal and professional implications of various paths in medicine is an important exercise to undertake early in one's career. It will aid in planning the stages of training and in ensuring personal and professional satisfaction with outcomes. Personal issues (e.g., illness or death of a family member) will arise unpredictably, and may alter one's intended training and career course. That being said, there can be many roads to the same goal.

Key references

Faulkner LR. 2007. Personal reflections on a career of transitions. *Journal of the American Academy of Psychiatry and the Law Online*. 35: 253–9.

Linzer M, Rosenberg M, McMurray JE, Glassroth J. 2002. Respecting the lifecycle: rational workforce planning for a section of general internal medicine. *American Journal of Medicine*. 113: 443–8.

A. Major transitions

Jordan Cohen, MD FRCPC

Objectives

This chapter will

- identify the key transitions that are made throughout a physician's career, and
- explore the challenges that may occur during these transitions.

> **Case**
> Residents in your program have identified a strong need for career counselling at an early stage of their education. They have pointed out that the lack of this resource contributes to their stress, decreases their sense of well-being and may lead them to make suboptimal choices in planning their training.

Introduction

All physicians go through the natural process of starting training as novice medical students and moving steadily toward becoming medical experts. Such transitions are a natural part of medical practice and continue throughout the medical life cycle. Learning to make transitions a time for reflection and mastery can be a valuable way to cultivate individual and professional resiliency.

Key life-cycle transitions

Transition to residency. For some trainees, the transition from medical school to residency is jarring and uncomfortable. For most, it is exciting, unnerving and deeply rewarding. Overnight, trainees are suddenly called "doctor," have a licence to practise medicine, begin to supervise medical students, and work reasonably independently from their supervisors. However, the learning curve is steep, and professional growth rapid. Many medical schools recognize that this transition can be stressful and have begun to develop special educational training programs (e.g., workshops on teaching/supervising, sessions on interprofessional collaboration, information sessions summarizing community resources and partnerships, lectures on medical error and ethics) to help trainees negotiate this change with ease.

Transition to practice. One model of the transition from residency to medical practice suggests that it unfolds in four phases (Misiaszek and Potter 1989):

1. **Termination**: grief over the loss of the residency,
2. **Adjustment:** ambivalence about the new role,
3. **Identity:** growth and development of new competence and the integration of commitment to lifelong learning and professional development, and
4. **Consolidation:** reaping the rewards of lifelong learning efforts and the acquisition of skills.

The early transition into practice requires a great deal of professional mentorship and personal support. Financial matters need to be considered carefully (e.g., retirement plans, insurance policies, power of attorney, will and testament, incorporation issues, contractual issues), professional matters need to be negotiated (e.g., assigned clinical duties, procurement of office space and administrative support, on-call duties), academic appointments settled (e.g., academic rank, career path, levels and types of supervision), and professional development strategies developed (e.g., identification of mentors, selection of CME courses, identification of knowledge gaps). New practitioners are strongly encouraged to recognize that they will benefit from help in each of these areas.

Transition to retirement

Perhaps the most critical issue in this phase of the physician life cycle is psychological readiness for retirement. Some physicians carefully and thoughtfully phase themselves into retirement with a clear idea of what their post-professional life will be like. Others suddenly stop practice. In general, experts on retirement strongly encourage physicians to take the former approach; the latter is most often associated with restlessness, boredom, dissatisfaction and regret.

Retirement also entails practical issues (financial, clinical, corporate, personal, family-related) that can be clarified with professional input and advice. Again, physicians are encouraged to plan, to use all resources open to them, and to move forward mindful of the fact they are in the middle of a significant life transition.

Normal life transitions

Along the way, physicians will also experience many life transitions, such as starting and ending relationships, accepting or ending specific jobs and roles, the birth and death of loved ones, and aspects of aging. As with all aspects of life, flexibility, mindfulness and support will make these transitions easier. Having a close network of friends, colleagues, advisors and mentors will promote resilience along the way.

Key references

CMA Centre for Physician Health and Well-being. 2004. The non-financial aspects of physician retirement: Environmental scan & literature review. Ottawa: Canadian Medical Association.

Misiaszek J and RL Potter. 1984. Transition from residency training to academia. *Psychiatric Quarterly*. 56 (3): 209–14.

Prince K, Van de Wiel M, Van der Vleuten C, Boshuizen H, Scherpbier A. 2004. Junior doctors' opinions about the transition from medical school to clinical practice: a change of environment. *Education for Health*. 17: 323–31.

Case resolution

At a departmental retreat, residents make a formal request for a mentoring and career counselling program. The faculty are supportive of this request and note that they would also benefit from the same sort of resource. The department chair and the program director agree to work with the university and its affiliated hospitals to create such a resource.

Key aspects of the mentoring program include

- biannual individual career planning sessions between leaders and mentees (e.g., program director and residents, chair and faculty, chair and dean),
- ongoing protected time for formal mentoring by all,
- identification of skilled mentors for mentees to consider (including practising and retired members of the department),
- annual workshops on mentoring (how to be a mentor and how to be a mentee),
- annual career days (focused on various models of practice and career development),
- annual sessions on academic promotion,
- annual workshops focused on the development of teaching and/or research skills, and
- fostering a culture of personal and professional support, including formal recognition (award programs) and informal celebration (rituals such as annual summer retreats, holiday dinners and spring barbeques).

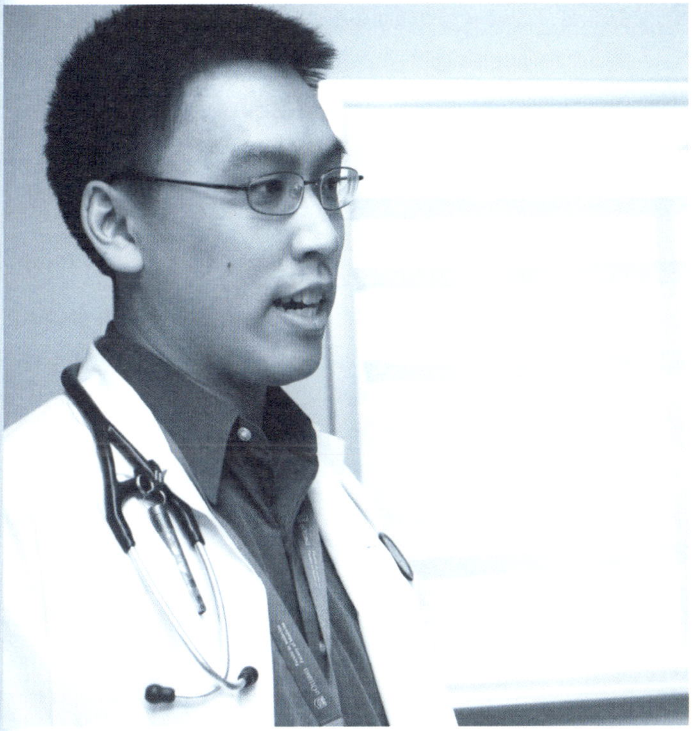

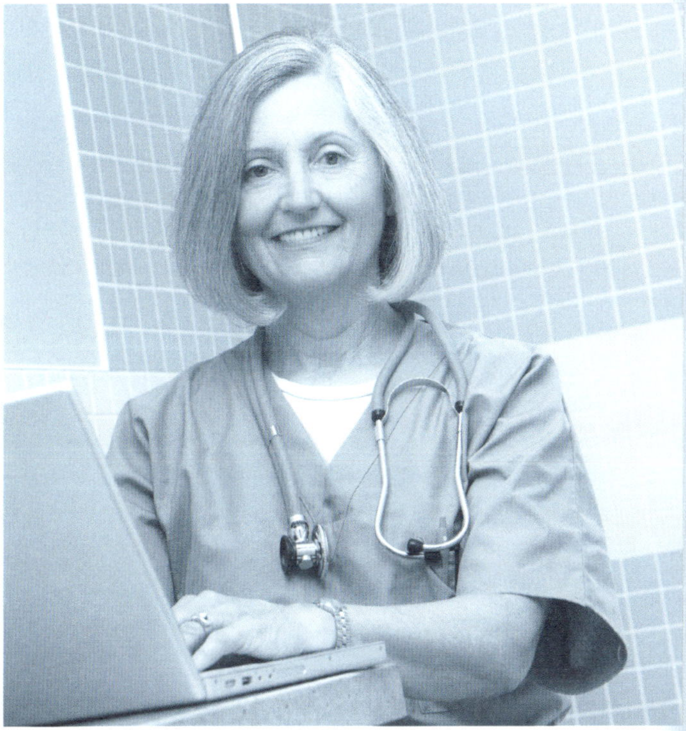

B. The importance of the practice and learning environment

Leslie Flynn, MD MMus CCFP FRCPC

Objectives

This chapter will

- identify facets of the health care work environment that shape physicians' professional and personal satisfaction,
- propose an approach to selecting a practice setting that best suits one's interests and needs, and
- discuss how, in any practice setting, physicians must be prepared to adapt to change.

Case

A resident is in the second year of residency. The more the resident engages in clinical practice, the more they find themselves concerned about the environments in which health care is delivered. Many of the resident's colleagues, other health professionals, and administrative staff seem frustrated and in various phases of burnout. Personally, the resident finds time spent with patients and supervisors to be sustaining, but the resident wonders if they will be able to tolerate "the system" over time. The resident wonders if they made the right career decision and, in spite of a love for clinical medicine, is considering shifting away from clinical practice. The resident mentions this to the chief resident, who listens thoughtfully and suggests bringing the matter up with their program director.

Introduction

One of the great joys, and one of the great challenges, of the practice of medicine is its incredibly rapid pace of change. Advances in biomedical knowledge are being made at an unprecedented pace. Technological innovations are transforming the manner in which patient investigations are conducted and care is delivered. Ongoing debates surrounding health care reform, together with shifting patient expectations, make for a challenging and often uncertain environment.

This rapid evolution comes at a price. Health care costs, paid for largely from the public purse, continue to rise exponentially. New models of management are under constant revision across Canada, and a consensus is growing that our health care system cannot continue to be sustained without significant reform. Hundreds of thousands of Canadians do not have a primary care provider, hospitals struggle to maintain nurses and physicians, emergency rooms are overcrowded, and wait times continue to get longer. Consequently, services are being redesigned, the roles of professionals are being revised, and funding is being frozen or reallocated. This is a time of great concern for Canada's universal health care system.

These challenges have exacerbated the stressors already inherent in the work of a physician. Demanding workloads and schedules, being in the near-constant presence of suffering, and struggling to find sufficient time for family and friends are no longer the only stressors within the health care environment. Indeed, for all health professionals, it can be a challenge to maintain a positive outlook and a healthy morale.

If not well managed, these stressors can lead to problematic behaviours. Sarcasm, gossip, cynicism, protectionism and withdrawal can all become an ingrained part of the health work environment. Morale suffers, while a genuine desire for collaborative and innovative practice begins to wane. Frustration rises, and professionals begin to feel that they have little input into or control over their practice and practice setting. A culture of blame and shame begins to form, making the work environment toxic. Tragically, such struggles are not uncommon in Canada.

Thankfully, we all have a role to play in contributing to a more positive health care work environment. Governments, professional organizations, training systems, hospitals and universities are all dedicated to the goal of stabilizing and strengthening Canada's health care system. There is much reason to have hope in the future.

Choosing wisely

On the level of the individual career, what is a physician to do? Although the current situation may seem dire, physicians should recognize the many choices that lie before them. These include the selection of specialty, the nature and location of their practice, and even the hours of work. If these choices have already been made, it is still possible to use positive strategies to optimize one's work environment.

Choosing a specialty requires consideration of many factors. Giving careful thought to the questions listed in the textbox may be of help.

Choosing a career path: Some factors to consider

- Do you require significant leisure time to maintain a sense of well-being?
- Do you prefer to work in teams, or alone?
- Does involvement in emergency care appeal to you?
- Do you want to work in hospital-based care?
- Do you want to be engaged in research, teaching and/or administration?

It is also wise to consider carefully one's preferences for practice setting. For example, although certain specialties can be practised only in a hospital setting, that hospital might be a community hospital situated in a small town or a large urban tertiary care centre. It might be an academic health sciences centre with a dedicated focus on teaching and research, or it might have no university affiliation and hence no mandate as a teaching centre. If a hospital setting is not necessary or is unappealing, there are ample opportunities to establish a solo or a group practice focused on ambulatory care. A group practice could be made up solely of physicians, or could include multiple health care disciplines in a team-based model of care. There are also opportunities for physicians to develop a career outside the clinical realm, at any stage in their career. Politics, the pharmaceutical industry, hospital management, insurance companies, health policy consultancies, and research and medical writing firms are all examples of the opportunities that exist, possibly after additional education in areas such as business management or public administration.

Consideration should also be given to the philosophy and tone of the workplace. It is essential to join an organization whose goals and vision are consistent with one's own values and aspirations. Does the organization's culture reflect what you think and believe? Is it compatible with your approach to life and patient care? This very important aspect of choosing a practice setting can be forgotten in the heat of negotiating dollars, space and operating room time.

Finally, do existing staff members appear to be happy? Are they a collegial group who appear to collaborate and to be respectful of each other? Notice how they interact with and address one other. An important element of sustaining pleasure in one's work is working with people who inspire trust and are committed to the work. There is clear evidence that health care environments with a positive atmosphere and are supportive of staff, recognizing all employees as assets, produce happier, healthier employees and more satisfied patients.

Because selecting a permanent place for one's practice requires the unhurried consideration of many factors, many people try a variety of practice settings before making a final decision. This can be done by choosing to do locums for a period of time after completion of training. This provides an opportunity to try a practice setting and its location on for size. Immersing oneself in a few different practice settings can lead to a discovery of what combination of features will best satisfy one's individual needs.

Coping with change

The health care work environment is never static, and regardless of where one practises there will always be challenges to face. Because change is a stressor, particularly when it is paired with uncertainty, we must anticipate that it can affect the work environment in a negative way. When this occurs, we need effective coping strategies.

Approaches that physicians can use to improve their current work environment include identifying problems clearly and objectively, discussing these problems with others in a way that expresses feelings but refrains from simply complaining and blaming, and proposing potential solutions. Offering to be part of a solution and contributing to the workplace with a positive attitude provides role modelling for all health care colleagues. Physicians seek to provide excellent clinical care to patients in an environment that is collegial, collaborative and personally satisfying. They can be instrumental to creating and sustaining positive work environments for the benefit of patients and of the entire health care team.

Case resolution

The resident meets with their program director of student affairs, who presents information regarding the many choices and opportunities that are available to specialty physicians. Together they consider career choices with respect to specialty and practice setting. They consider how to approach the work environment that the resident is currently finding challenging. The resident selects a mentor to help them learn how to manage system issues and begins to feel more hopeful about their future practice.

Key references

Lindström K. 1994. Psychosocial criteria for good work organization. *Scandinavian Journal of Work, Environment & Health*. 20: 123-33.

Sotile WM, Sotile MO. 2002. *The Resilient Physician: Effective Emotional Management for Doctors and Their Medical Organizations*. Chicago: American Medical Association.

C. Career planning: The early stages

Meridith Marks, MD FRCPC

Objectives

This chapter will

- outline the importance of career planning throughout the medical lifecycle, and
- summarize five common themes involved in early career planning.

> **Case**
>
> A resident is quickly moving through residency and generally loves everything about medicine—procedures, clinics, research, teaching, community care, etc. In fact, the resident is feeling anxious about the pending sub-specialty decision. On one hand, the resident wants to keep all of their options open. On the other hand, the resident recognizes that a more narrow focus may be in order to plan the next phase of their career. The resident just doesn't quite know what to do.

Introduction

For many residents, focusing on completing medical school and then residency can leave little room to consider how their career might unfold after they have completed their certification examinations. However, career planning should start early during residency, since decisions made at this stage will have a significant impact on subsequent career directions. At the same time, it is important to keep one's options—and mind—open. Many residents change their plans as they move through residency and experience different areas of practice. The ideal job might not be available when one is ready for it, and so it is important to be prepared to work toward one's career objectives over time.

Early career planning questions

Academic versus private practice. One of the first questions residents often consider in planning their career path is whether they would prefer to work in an academic or a private practice. In reality, these two options are not mutually exclusive. The term academic practice usually refers to a practice affiliated with an academic health sciences centre and that requires an academic appointment with a university. It carries with it an expectation to contribute to the education of medical students and residents and to make a contribution to medical scholarship. Most physicians interested in pursuing research will opt for an academic practice. Typically, academic practices are group practices and operate under a range of remuneration models, ranging from set salaries to fee-for-service billing. Alternatively, a practice plan may be in place to distribute the income of a group on the basis of patient caseload and academic activities.

The term private practice usually implies that one's primary practice is located independently of a hospital or a faculty of medicine. One is paid on a fee-for-service basis and is responsible for all expenses associated with running one's own office. Indeed, setting up a private practice is not unlike starting a business. Many physicians report that they are ill-prepared for this aspect when they first start practice. Seeking financial advice before setting up such a practice is well advised. Although this is not a requirement, many private practitioners also have an affiliation or part-time academic appointment with a medical school, and thus contribute to the education of students and residents. Depending on the medical school, a stipend may be associated with these affiliations.

Hospital versus community-based practice. It is certainly possible to combine hospital and community-based practices, especially in non-academic settings and smaller communities. Many physicians with a community office have hospital privileges. Continuity of care and the variety of one's practice is typically greater in such situations. However, such arrangements also mean having to balance one's work day to meet multiple demands.

Some physicians provide care in only one setting, often because of a focus on primary or secondary care. For example, community-based pediatricians, family physicians and psychiatrists who do not admit patients to hospital work exclusively in a primary care setting, while those who provide tertiary care can be solely hospital-based. The type of patients cared for, the needs of specific communities, and professional and personal desires all influence career decisions in this regard.

Specialized versus general practice. Within family medicine and the Royal College specialties there are varying degrees of specialization. A general surgeon may sub-specialize in irritable bowel disease, while a family physician may focus on care of the elderly. Alternatively, some family physicians are the only medical practitioner in small communities. The focus of one's practice may well dictate other characteristics of that practice. It is important for residents to remember that although they may desire a sub-specialized practice, it can take some time for such a practice to be developed. It is always prudent to be prepared for all aspects of practice; one never knows what opportunities may lie ahead.

Group versus solo practice. True solo practices are now increasingly rare as group practices become the norm. There can be considerable variability between group practices. Some simply share infrastructure and expenses, while others share the care of patients. Other group practices are now interdisciplinary in nature. For example, one may find an orthopedic surgeon, a neurosurgeon and a physiatrist working together in a specialized clinic.

Although most academic practices are affiliated with a group, in some situations a single specialist provides care for a specific patient population. For example, a single physician in a practice devoted to gastrointestinal disease might provide a procedure that requires specific expertise, such as endoscopic retrograde cholangiopancreatography. In situations where a single physician provides a certain type of care, patients and some administrators may have unrealistic expectations about that practitioner's availability. In such cases it is especially important to consider how one's practice will be covered during times of illness, in the face of family responsibilities, or when it is time for a vacation.

Urban versus rural practice. The choice of an urban versus a rural setting dictates many other characteristics of a practice. Physicians in a rural practice are likely to be generalists and have an increased probability of working alone. Physicians in rural areas tend to like the diverse nature of their practice and the independence associated with it. At the same time, they need to be prepared to cope with limited resources and to recognize they may have to transfer some patients to tertiary care hospitals in an urban centre. By the same token, those who are interested in a highly specialized area of practice are likely to need the resources available only in large urban centres.

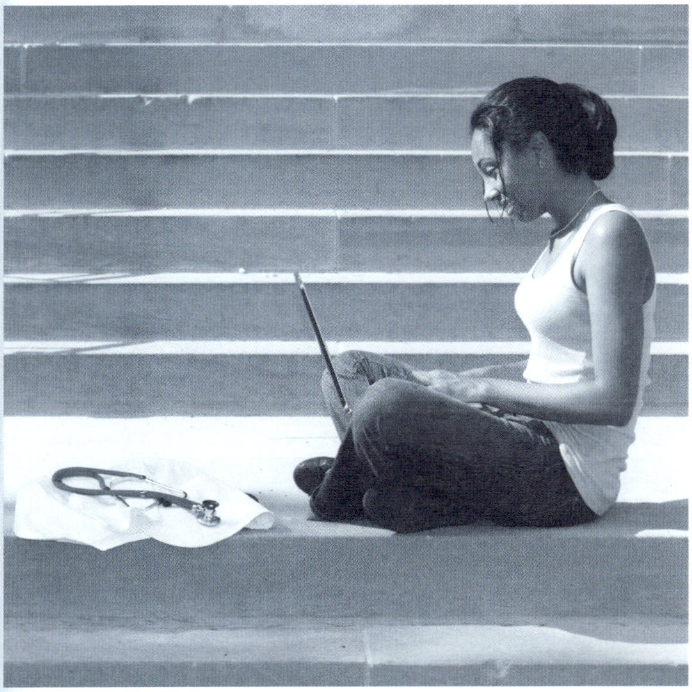

Do you really know what you want?

You may think you know as a resident what you want your future practice to look like, but do you really? Did you really know what was involved in being a medical student when you started medical school? Some aspects of practice need to be experienced to be understood. Doing electives and speaking with others in similar situations will help, but a month of being on-call in an ideal practice setting can be enough to confirm one's expectations—or to revise them entirely.

As one plans for potential electives, fellowships and advanced degree studies it is important to consider future practice goals from the various angles outlined here. But it is also important not to exclude too many options until you have tried out what you think might be right for you. Your ideal practice might turn out less interesting or rewarding than you imagine. Or you might discover an unexpected affinity for some other area. Remember, too, that life can take us in many directions: family responsibilities, opportunities, newly discovered passions, finances and health issues affect all of us in ways we do not foresee. Be prepared for varying practice possibilities during your career.

Case resolution

The resident meets with their mentor, the program director and a few recent graduates of the specialty program; informally over several months. The resident begins to appreciate that their skills fit an academic environment well, that they consider procedures an important part of practice, and that they would like to practice in a group setting. The resident makes a decision to sub-specialize in an interventional program with a clinical-investigator program, and begins to consider where they would like to build a practice after residency.

Key references

American Medical Association. *JAMA CareerNet: Networking for Physicians.* Last viewed on August 6, 2009: jamacareernet.ama-assn.org/

BMJ Publishing Group. *BMJ Careers.* Last viewed on August 6, 2009: careers.bmj.com/careers/hospital-medical-healthcare-jobs.html

McMillan J, Neligan P, Clegg D. 2009. Career planning is key for medical graduates. *Target Jobs.* Last viewed on August 6, 2009: targetjobs.co.uk/medicine/articleview-50s_34a_2253.aspx

D. Coping with change

Derek Puddester, MD MEd FRCPC

Objectives

This chapter will

- examine why change is associated with stress and distress,
- consider strategies for individuals to cope with and manage change, and
- propose strategies that teams of professionals can use to cope with and manage change.

> **Case**
>
> A fellow is looking forward to moving into an academic staff position at the end of their training. The fellow has been mentored by the department chair, enjoys healthy relationships with many of their colleagues, and is connected to the community in many ways.
>
> Late on a Friday afternoon, an email is sent to all members of the department noting that the chair has resigned and been replaced. The new chair has been recruited by the dean specifically to bring major change to the group. Research infrastructure is expected to double, all new specialists are expected to progress to the academic rank of associate professor within five years, and clinical services are set to increase by 25 per cent in three years.
>
> The fellow had hoped to build a clinical practice and has no particular interest in an academic career. The fellow's nicely planned career path seems to be threatened by change.

Introduction

One way to approach change is to determine where we are in the cycle of change. Picture a horizontal axis that measures participation in change and a vertical axis that measures acceptance of change. This creates a useful grid that can be considered with the help of a seafaring metaphor. In the first zone of change, people have a high acceptance of change and a high degree of participation in the change process: these are the crew. In the second zone, people have a high acceptance of change but low participation in the process: these are the passengers. In the third zone, people have a low acceptance of change and low participation in the change process: these are the cargo containers. In the fourth zone, people have a low acceptance of change but a high rate of participation: these are the pirates. A well-managed change process is mindful of all four roles, and a well-led process sails the ship through rough seas and reaches the destination unharmed (figure 4).

Strategies for dealing with change

Strategy 1: Know yourself. This guide stresses the importance of knowing one's self, one's values and one's beliefs. In the cycle of change, checking-in with these core aspects of ourselves can help us measure our responses to the change being demanded.

> The fellow starts here, carefully considering a feeling of shock at the sudden loss of a mentor and career plan, as well as the need for a career focused largely on clinical medicine.

Strategy 2: Review assumptions. Change can trigger significant anxiety. If physicians have a pessimistic, cynical or distrustful view of the world, they will likely find change threatening. If that view is expressed through negative coping strategies, such as aggression, catastrophic thinking or an impulse to sabotage the situation, then significant harm can result. Pirates rarely win, hurt others along the way, and end up in a place characterized by failure and isolation.

For physicians with an optimistic, flexible and positive world view, change can be energizing. Such a view coupled with positive coping strategies can lead to positive, innovative and synergistic outcomes. Crew members thrive as part of healthy teams, enjoy personal growth and development, and enjoy a destination characterized by success and connectivity.

> The fellow reviews some of their assumptions with care. First, the fellow realizes a deep distrust of the university's internal politics, given the abruptness of the mentor's departure. However, the fellow also realizes that they may not appreciate all the issues involved and that personal feelings may be clouding professional judgment. The fellow phones the mentor, only to discover that he is fully supportive of the change in leadership, as he is dealing with a terminal illness. He had planned to inform the fellow of this situation during their mentorship meeting early in the coming week.

Strategy 3: Seek supports. Whenever our defences are activated we are trying to protect ourselves from harm. These defences can be positive and constructive, but they can also cause us to deny the legitimacy of alternative perspectives, to misconstrue the truth, and to dismiss our own errors and vulnerabilities. Seeking the perspectives of others can provide a helpful corrective to one-sided perceptions. Friends and family members know us well and can often help us confront issues we might otherwise avoid. Colleagues can also serve in this role, particularly with respect to professional issues and situations.

Finally, if our own vulnerabilities are strong and our coping skills not particularly healthy, working with a professional (a life coach, mentor or therapist) can be of value.

> The fellow meets with the other fellows in the department and discovers that everyone is dealing with the news in a similar fashion. They openly discuss their concerns about job security, workplace culture, and the way in which information was either withheld or presented late in the change process. More importantly, they talk about the positive possibilities that the announced changes might bring. One of the fellows notes that enhanced academic activity might facilitate the development of new resources for clinical activity. The fellow begins to feel less distressed.

Figure 4: Coping with change grid - seafaring metaphor

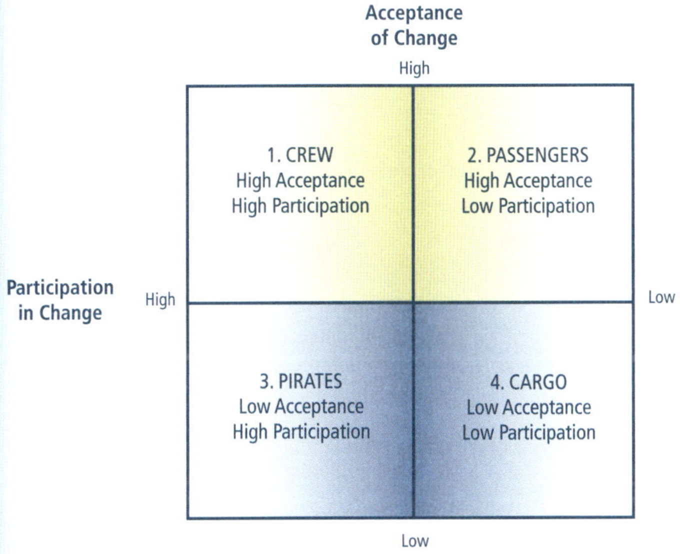

Strategy 4: Be flexible and anticipate the unexpected. When a hurricane hits landfall, the most vulnerable objects are those that are rigid. Without flexibility, structures cannot cope with stress and tend to snap or bend hopelessly out of shape. At the same time, resistance to change can be helpful in illustrating aspects of change that deserve review and further consideration. In practical terms, this means ensuring that we take time to carefully reflect on aspects of change, thinking of various ways we can and ought to react to circumstances, and being mindful of our habitual reactions and how they are perceived by others. Being open to alternatives, being careful to project genuine thoughtfulness and consideration, and avoiding knee-jerk reactions holds us in good stead.

> The fellow moves from a perspective of frank hostility toward the new chair to a stance that is at least open to considering how the fellow might fit within the department's new vision.

Strategy 5: Maintain perspective and balance. When the waves of change are high it can be difficult to remember that change goes through phases and that the storm will eventually wind down. When we are feeling consumed by change, it is critical to force ourselves to shift perspectives. Physical activity, mindful practices, healthy distraction, time with loved ones and good friends, and engagement in hobbies and activities take on more importance. These activities remove us from the stress of change and also help us put our worries in perspective.

> The fellow begins to spend more time at the gym, as working out helps clear their head and brings them new insights. One evening, the fellow develops a draft model of a new clinical service. Suddenly, they see how placing that model in an academic setting could create new and innovative opportunities. The fellow also begins to spend more time with their hockey team and enjoys the break that this activity gives from the work-related worries.

Strategy 6: Keep moving forward. Periods of intense change invariably come to a close. It can be helpful to consider where we would like to be at the end of that phase and to do what we can to progress toward that goal. If we allow ourselves to keep moving forward, and allow ourselves to be flexible and to let some things go, we are likely to end up in a better place than the one we left behind.

> ### Case resolution
> The fellow meets with the new chair and shares their personal career goals and aspirations. Together, they realize that a new opportunity in quality management exists that would allow the fellow to contribute to the academic mission of the department while focusing primarily on clinical practice. Several years later, the fellow is deeply satisfied with their clinical practice and overall position within the department.

Key references

Bridges W. 2003. *Managing Transitions: Making the Most of Change*. New York: Da Capo Press.

Flach F. 2009. *Choices: Coping Creatively with Personal Change*. New York: Hatherleigh Press.

Kotter JP. 1996. *Leading Change*. Cambridge: Harvard Business School Press.

Introduction: Physician health care needs: Unique issues

Derek Puddester, MD MEd FRCPC

Physician health is emerging as a unique field of clinical practice, scholarship and policy development. Initially, efforts in physician health focused largely on helping to recognize, treat and rehabilitate physicians with substance use disorders. Success in this area has led to an awareness that physicians also need help with mental health problems such as depression, anxiety and burnout. Our contemporary view is that physician health is a holistic and broad construct, that it is important to acknowledge the broad determinants of physician health, and that a greater focus is needed on the promotion of health and healthy behaviours among physicians and trainees.

The chapters in this section will outline a number of unique issues of importance to meeting the needs of Canada's physicians, as follows:

Physical health

This chapter will emphasize the importance for physicians of having a primary care provider, outline unique issues faced by physicians as patients and as health care providers for other physicians, and suggest practical strategies that can directly promote physicians' physical health.

Mental health

It is alarming to consider that the rate of suicide among medical professionals and trainees is much higher than among the general population. Fortunately, physicians and medical students are increasingly recognizing the importance of mental health, and physician health programs are reporting a rise in the number of requests received for help in this area. This section will outline the most common mental health issues among physicians, summarize the challenges physicians face when they consider or seek care, and emphasize how intervention and treatment are highly successful.

Substance use, abuse and dependence

Eight per cent of physicians will struggle with substance abuse and dependence at some point during their career. The consequences of substance dependence can be significant, and it can be challenging for family members, colleagues and patients to know how best to manage concerns they have about a physician's potential substance use. This chapter will outline practical strategies readers can use to recognize substance problems, offer suggestions on intervention, and summarize the positive prognosis associated with this class of disorders.

Caring for colleagues

It is essential that physicians have access to clinical services that appreciate the unique aspects of care associated with physician health. This chapter is designed to help inform providers on issues that require particular attention, such as establishing rapport, boundaries, confidentiality and privacy.

Mandatory reporting

Perhaps the most confusing and uncomfortable area of concern to physicians as patients, and to physicians providing care to other physicians, is mandatory reporting. This chapter outlines some of the key principles involved in mandatory reporting, offers practical tips and strategies to inform the decision to report (or not), and suggest further resources that physicians may consult.

Physician health programs

Canada has a national network of physician health programs that allows every medical student, resident and practising physician access to services and programs focused on their unique health needs. This chapter summarizes the history of these programs, outlines other national efforts in physician health such as educational programs, position statements and research activities, and directs readers to resources they can access on a local or national level.

Stress and coping

This chapter highlights the insights gleaned from a survey of a large sample of Canadian specialists on normal patterns of stress and coping. Key aspects of resiliency are summarized as well as several of the unique sources of stress in the medical workplace.

Physicians with an illness or disability

There is remarkably little in the literature about physicians who become ill or disabled during their training or practice. However, it is essential that such physicians have access to quality rehabilitative services, appropriate accommodations, and reasonable opportunities to serve the public. This section will address these themes and outline other resources that readers can use.

There is no doubt that many other facets of health and sustainability are of relevance to physicians. Many other sections of the Physician Health Guide will be of value in your search for information and practical ways to move forward with your own personal health and professional sustainability strategy.

Key references

- **www.ephysicianhealth.com** This free and anonymous online resource was written and designed by Canadian experts in physician health. Interactive and practical, it includes sections on relationships, depression and anxiety, resiliency, substance use, personal care and many other issues.
- **www.eworkplacehealth.com** Also a free and anonymous online resource, this program focuses on the needs of health professionals in the workplace. Offering interactive exercises focused on the development of insight and skills, it blends many of the skills of this section of the guide and offers practical methods to enhance the health care workplace.
- **www.cma.ca** The Canadian Medical Association's *Centre for Physician Health and Well-being* offers a rich clearinghouse of reference material on physician health, information on upcoming conferences and workshops, and additional learning resources on physician health.

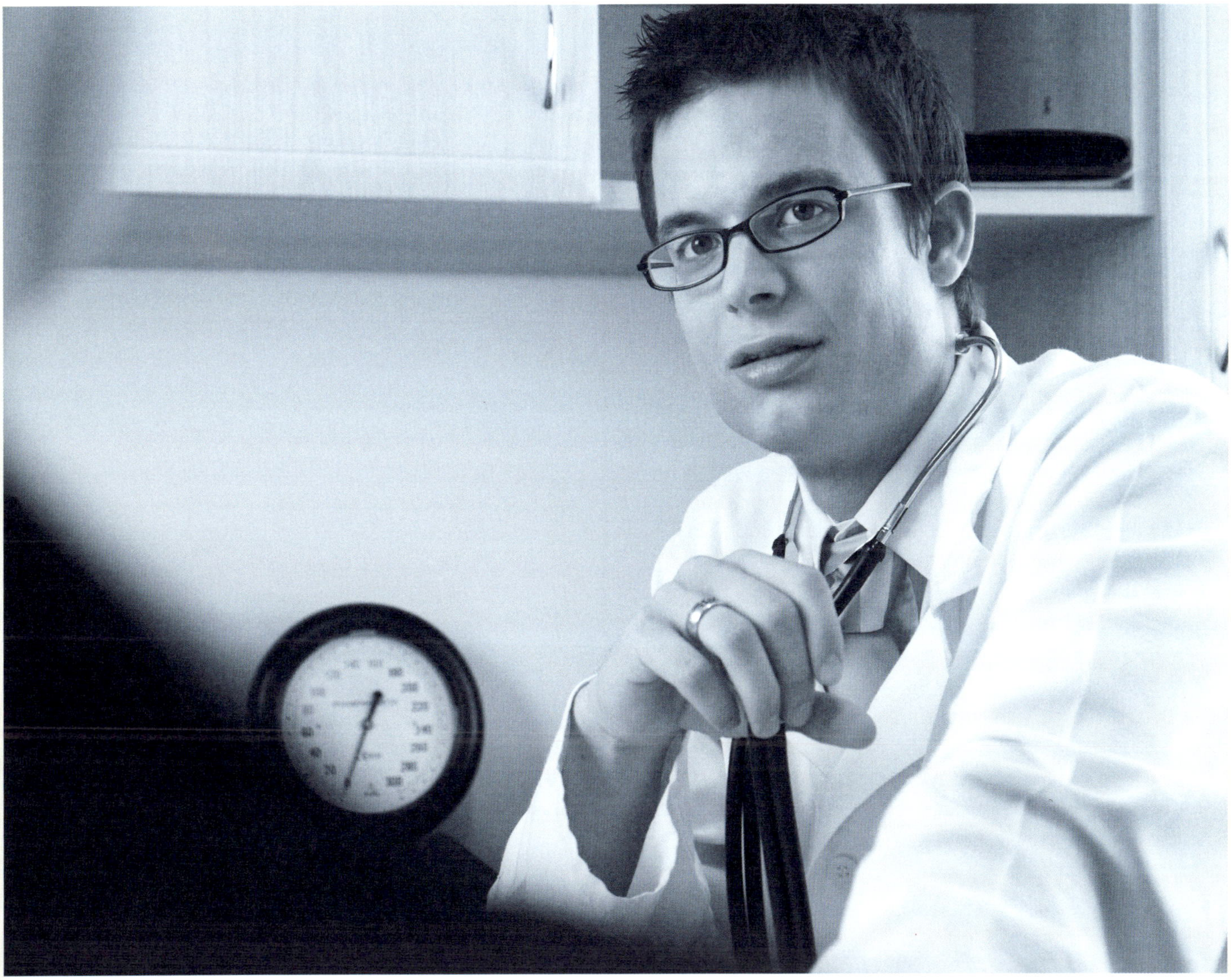

A. Physical health

Lee Donohue, MD MHSc

Objectives

This chapter will

- outline preventive care guidelines,
- discuss age-appropriate screening and prevention, and
- describe methodological problems in researching the physical health of physicians.

> **Case**
>
> A fourth-year resident has planned a dream vacation with their spouse to Africa. The spouse is concerned that the resident keeps putting off getting vaccinations and has indicated that the trip will be cancelled unless the resident meets with their family physician and takes care of this responsibility. Frustrated, the resident turns to a fellow in infectious disease and asks for help, as the resident feels too busy to see a family physician.

Introduction

Physicians receive care that is different from that obtained by other people because they are "physician patients." To expect a physician patient to behave like a patient without medical training is unrealistic. To expect a treating physician to provide generic medical care and ignore occupational issues specific to physicians is also unrealistic. Physicians have a high level of medical knowledge, a high level of access to health information and, generally, a high level of self-care. It is not known how physicians apply their knowledge and experience to decisions about their own medical care. Although physicians have had extensive training, they may lack information on prevention, screening, diagnosis and treatments in certain areas.

The underuse of family physicians and preventive health services by physicians themselves is notable and concerning. In general, physicians have the same physical health problems as the rest of the population. In some cases, they are in better health (e.g., they smoke less and exercise more); in other respects they are at higher risk (e.g., of suicide and substance use). Periodic health examinations may be the only consultation with a health professional that physician patients receive. Although some health economists maintain that an annual review is not an efficient use of health care resources, patients and physicians generally agree that this review can strengthen the physician–patient relationship. The average patient has three to six visits with their family physicians annually, and almost 80 per cent of preventive care advice is received during non-preventive visits. Physician patients, even those with health problems or concerns, likely have far fewer routine visits than the average patient; thus, a periodic health examination is of great importance to this group.

Quality indicators are rarely reported in the few studies of physicians' physical health. Yizchak Dresner examined population quality indicators for physicians as compared to non physicians. Among patients with hypertension, 56 per cent of those who were physician patients had their blood pressure monitored, as compared with 77 per cent of those who were members of the general population. Screening colonoscopy rates were higher and fecal occult blood testing rates lower among physicians. For complex reasons, it appears that the care physician patients receive is not equivalent to that of others. This is not always to their advantage.

Unique issues for physician patients and their providers

All patients self-diagnose, including physician patients. And, as with all patients who self-diagnose, one risk of doing so is that it can lead to delays in obtaining necessary care. Like other patients, a physician patient may fail to recognize the seriousness of a symptom or to recognize non-specific symptoms. And, like others, physician patients may avoid seeking care because of embarrassment and concerns about confidentiality.

Physician patients also have a tendency to edit out information that does not fit with their original self-diagnosis. This clinical certainty may be unwarranted. A personal physician caring for you, a physician patient, will consider what you know, what you think you know, what you would like to know, and what you need to know in order to manage your health care.

> **Preparing for a primary care visit: Tips for the physician patient**
>
> - Book an appointment and advise the staff of the issues you would like to discuss so that sufficient time can be allocated to you.
> - Bring a family member: other patients do.
> - Make a list of concerns to share with your physician.
> - Prioritize your list.
> - Bring in all your prescription and nonprescription medications, including samples of medications.
> - Bring copies of tests that you or others have ordered.
> - Take notes during your appointment.
> - If you need to cancel, call and rebook immediately.
> - Schedule a periodic health examination.

Summary

Family physicians are specialists who have a critical role to play in sustaining the health of fellow health professionals, including physicians. Because physicians have both normal and unique health care needs, it is important for all to seek out and appropriately utilize a family physician.

Case resolution

The fellow gently and respectfully refuses to treat the resident. The fellow suggests that the resident see a family physician, as it has been three years since the last primary care visit. Together they review the resident's schedule to find a time when the resident can slip away without compromising patient care or educational demands. The resident sees the family physician and begins a series of vaccinations. During the appointment, the resident is surprised to learn that their weight has gone up by 15 pounds. This leads to a conversation about some other important health concerns. The resident receives counselling about weight management, agrees to complete the recommended screening tests for their age and books a follow-up appointment.

Key references

Dresner Y. 2008. Do doctors look after their health as well as their patients? Results from the quality indicators program in our district. Presented at *2008 BMA—AMA—CMA International Conference on Doctors' Health: Doctors' Health Matters—Finding the Balance.* November 2008.

Tyssen R. 2007. Health problems and the use of health services among physicians: A review article with particular emphasis on Norwegian studies. *Industrial Health.* 45: 599-610.

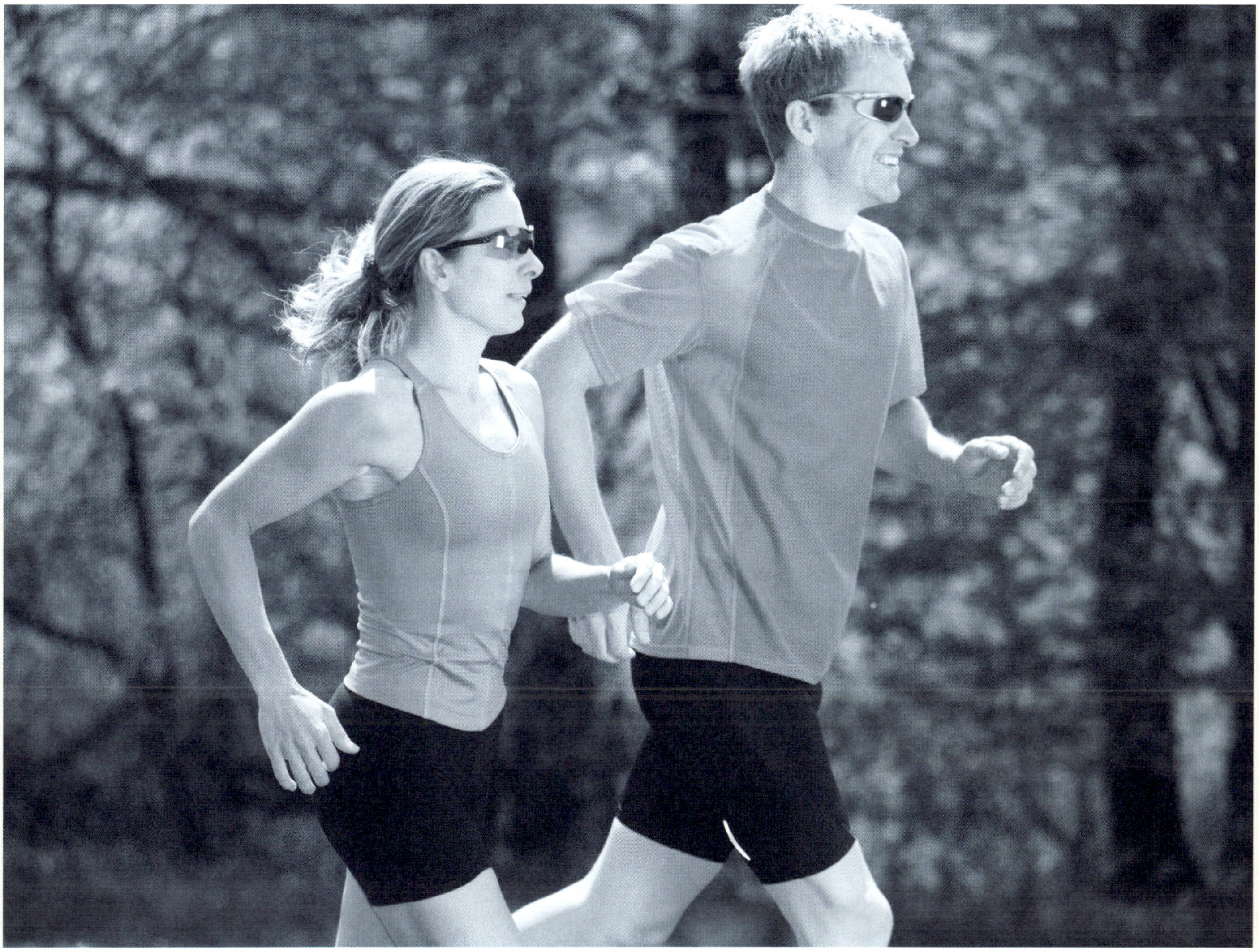

B. Mental health issues

Joy Albuquerque, MD MA FRCPC

Objectives

This chapter will

- discuss the prevalence of psychiatric illness, including suicidality, among physicians, and
- examine the importance for physicians of identifying signs and symptoms of serious emotional distress in themselves and in their colleagues.

> **Case**
>
> A first-year resident is paged to the delivery room because a patient they are following has gone into labour. This is the resident's first high-risk delivery and the resident is both excited and nervous. As the resident jogs toward the delivery suite they become aware of an uncomfortable feeling in the back of their neck and the pit of their stomach. The resident suddenly notices that they are having difficulty catching their breath and is experiencing chest pain. Fear engulfs the resident. A nurse notices the resident's difficulty and takes them to the emergency department. After full investigation, the episode is deemed to have been an anxiety attack. The resident is mortified that this has happened and is humiliated by what people must think. Even more terrifying is the thought that this could happen to them again. Everyone around the resident assures them that this panic occurred because of a combination of having been on call, not sleeping well and having missed lunch, and that the resident would be just fine.

Introduction

Mental health issues ranging from mild distress to severe and disabling psychiatric syndromes are among the leading causes of disability in the general population. For example, the point prevalence of major depressive disorder in the general population is approximately seven per cent. Studies suggest that rates of mood and anxiety disorders are slightly lower among working physicians, but research also shows that serious emotional distress is not rare in the physician population. Indeed, a meta-analysis found that female physicians are three times more likely to commit suicide than members of the general female population, while the suicide rate among male physicians is 1.4 times higher than among the general male population.

Among the factors known to contribute to physician stress are their high-pressure training and practice environments, the challenging decisions they must make every day, long and irregular work hours, and constantly witnessing sickness and impairment. In addition, some personality traits such as perfectionism, a tendency to assume responsibility for events, a strong work ethic and a robust desire to help others can contribute to the risk of emotional distress and mental illness.

Recognizing mental health problems among physicians

Emotional distress and mental illness tends to be under-detected among physicians. Many psychiatric disorders have a detrimental effect on a person's sense of self-efficacy and confidence, and it is not a stretch to imagine why doctors would conceal their psychological problems. For example, a depressed physicians, beset by guilt, may be impelled to work harder and longer hours to make up for perceived shortcomings. Because terms like stress, burnout and anxiety are so much a part of the usual banter in the medical world, physicians may use them to gloss over warning signals such as persistent worries, irritability, concentration problems and insomnia until those symptoms become disabling. Often, physicians with mental health difficulties present with compensatory behaviours such as self-medication, alcohol or drug abuse.

Risk factors for mental illness in the general population, including family history and previous episodes of psychiatric illness apply to medical students, residents and physicians. Education about these factors needs to occur early in a physician's training.

> **Key points: physicians and mental illness**
>
> - Physicians have the same vulnerabilities to mental illness as the general population.
> - Physicians running into psychological difficulty tend to mask it, behaving as if they were invulnerable.
> - Take seriously a colleague who shows signs of depression.
> - Suicide is a real problem, and doctors who have suicidal ideation need care urgently.
> - Education and behavioural adjustments are necessary to improve the ability to cope with the stresses of a medical career and to enhance personal resilience.

Another challenge faced by doctors with psychiatric disorders is a fear of being stigmatized or marginalized by the profession. Such fear can present as apprehensions about losing one's livelihood, being rejected by colleagues and patients, the possibility of regulatory sanctions, and generally diminished career options. Serious, recurrent mental health problems can change one's professional life and affect work performance and patient safety. Working on-call, typical or heroic hours, or performing in complex clinical environments might eventually, for some doctors with disabling mood disorders, become a thing of the past.

Given the safety-sensitive work of physicians, it is important that they obtain appropriate treatment when they are ill; unfortunately, an attitude of invincibility can pose a significant barrier to this. By extension, physicians who do reach out for help need to be taken seriously by their colleagues. However, corridor consultations and collegial interventions, even with the best intentions, can result in inaccurate diagnoses and sub-optimal treatment. It is essential that appropriate boundaries between the physician provider and the physician patient be established and respected.

Approximately 70 to 90 per cent of suicides are associated with mental illness. Given physicians' unique familiarity with death and their ready access to lethal means, suicide in this population is a serious issue. If a colleague expresses suicidal ideation or a sense of hopelessness it is vital to connect him or her to help expeditiously—whether to a personal physician, psychiatrist or emergency service. It is important not to downgrade the clinical concern because the person is a physician. Those who treat physicians with depression need to carefully probe for suicidal intent and to treat the illness aggressively.

Improving personal resiliency can help physicians cope with the myriad of problems and stressors in a life in medicine. Insisting on reasonable work hours and workload, exercising regularly and taking time for friends and family are essential. However, mental illness cannot be entirely prevented. Although it is difficult to predict the first onset of a mood disorder, physicians who have recovered from an episode should consider their exposure to triggers, including shift work, and explore evidence-based prevention strategies.

Early detection, education and treatment of mental health disorders are crucial in this safety sensitive profession. Appropriate follow-up and monitoring of these conditions, particularly those that recur, is essential for physicians with mental illness not only as individuals but also as professionals who wish to safely and competently practise their chosen vocation.

Case resolution

The resident speaks to their family physician, who organizes a mental health assessment by a psychologist. The resident discloses a longstanding history of anxiety that has typically been ignored or minimized. The resident realizes that they are vulnerable to panic and anxiety when sleep-deprived, not eating well, socially isolated or under significant academic pressure. The resident agrees to a trial of therapy and learns better skills of self-care, relaxation and mindfulness. Slowly, the symptoms wane and the resident enjoys much better health, self-awareness and growing sense of confidence.

Key references

Fahrenkopf AM, Sectish TC, Barger LK, Sharek PJ, Lewin D, Chiang VW, et al. 2008. Rates of medication errors among depressed and burnt out residents: prospective cohort study. *BMJ*. 336 (7642): 488–91

Myers MF and GO Gabbard. 2008. *The Physician as Patient: A Clinical Handbook for Mental Health Professionals*. Arlington: American Psychiatric Publishing.

Schernhammer ES and GA Colditz. 2004. Suicide rates among physicians: A quantitative and gender assessment. *American Journal of Psychiatry*. 161 (12): 2295–302.

C. Substance use, abuse and dependence

Michael Kaufmann, MD (Dip)ABAM FCFP

Objectives

This chapter will

- discuss the nature and prevalence of substance use disorders as they affect physicians,
- describe signs of substance abuse in physicians, and
- present an approach to helping substance-abusing colleagues get the help they need.

> **Case**
>
> A resident is completing a fellowship and is in their final year. The resident has struggled academically during the fellowship because of marital problems, financial difficulties, and worries about ill parents. Over the past year, the resident has noticed that they have taken to drinking daily after work. In the past two months, this alcohol use has increased and the resident has begun to keep a flask in their work locker. One of the resident's close colleagues begins to suspect alcohol abuse when she notices the resident slurring words during afternoon handover and smells alcohol on the resident's breath.

Introduction

Medical students, residents and physicians are as human as their patients. They experience substance use disorders just as others do. In North America since the 1970s, the medical profession has acknowledged this fact and understood that substance use disorders are a health problem. An important facet of addressing the issue is learning how to recognize substance use problems in medical colleagues, intervening on their behalf, and directing them to the excellent treatment resources that do exist. Rehabilitation with careful, long-term follow-up and monitoring is more constructive than a punitive, disciplinary approach.

Substance use disorders in physicians

Neither epidemic nor inconsequential, the prevalence of serious substance abuse and dependence in physicians is in the region of eight per cent (Hughes 1992). This means that, over the course of a lifetime in practice, nearly one doctor in 10 will experience a problem with drug or alcohol abuse or dependence that will have a significant and potentially serious impact upon their lives and the lives of others around them. Alcohol is the most common drug of choice for doctors, followed by opioids and other substances.

It is important to view substance dependence as a chronic primary disorder that, without treatment, can be progressive and even fatal. Substance abuse is not the same as dependence. It is characterized by a pattern of maladaptive use of substance(s) that interferes with health and/or quality of life. This diagnosis can be made if criteria for substance dependence are not met. Substance abuse can progress to dependence if it is not addressed. Expert assessment, including clinical history, physical examination, lab and toxicology studies and collateral history, is often needed to formulate an accurate diagnosis.

Risk factors

Physicians probably experience substance use disorders at much the same rate as the general population. Although they don't have risks associated with low socio-economic status, there are other risks especially associated with being a physician. It has been postulated that many physicians have personality traits that contribute both to their professional success and to their personal vulnerability. They are compassionate people, dedicated in the extreme to the well-being of their patients, even at the expense of their own basic health needs. They tend to have perfectionistic and obsessive personality traits. They are often rigidly self-controlled. Stressed, and lacking healthy personal coping strategies, some find ease and comfort in the use of drugs or alcohol.

Access to drugs and the pharmacological optimism that comes with expert experience in prescribing for patients opens the door to drug self-administration. Anesthesiologists who inject themselves with potent opioids such as fentanyl, which are particularly prone to cause dependency, are a special case that illustrates this point.

Physicians who are experiencing substance abuse problems seldom receive assistance early in the course of their illness. They deny the magnitude of the problem, just as others—in their discomfort and uncertainty about how to help—deny what they are observing. They fear that reaching out for help might result in a report to their training program or to regulatory or other authorities, leading to the end of their career, livelihood and sense of self. They are needlessly trapped in their fear and shame. Meanwhile, the bystanders who do nothing become part of the problem.

Recognition

There is rarely a single observation that will clearly identify a substance-abusing colleague, at least not early in the progression of their illness. Physicians are skilled at presenting an appearance of calm and self-control even when they are suffering. Sensitive to the shame and stigma that are often attached to these problems, affected physicians will go to great lengths to conceal their disorder from colleagues, even when they are no longer able to disguise their problems at home. But some clues can be readily apparent to a caring colleague, especially if they are familiar with the doctor's baseline behaviour and personality (see textbox).

Signs of substance abuse or dependence in physicians

- mood swings and/or irritability,
- loss of efficiency and reliability,
- a decline in standards of dress and grooming,
- increased somatic complaints, illness and fatigue,
- increasing personal and professional isolation,
- unpredictable and irregular work habits and patterns,
- in residents, a drop-off in academic performance,
- delays in answering pages,
- increasing absenteeism, being "missing in action" and frequent bathroom breaks,
- angry outbursts resulting in staff and patient complaints,
- deterioration in handwriting and charting,
- inappropriate prescribing of large amounts of narcotics,
- heavy use of alcohol at staff social and CME events,
- heavy wastage of drugs and inappropriate drug handling,
- alcohol on the breath at work,
- nodding off at work,
- being caught drinking or self-administering drugs at work,
- therapeutic error or mishap, and
- suicidal gesturing.

Intervention

Waiting until a physician with a substance use problem asks for help, if that time ever comes, can have tragic results. We must pay attention to signs of distress in our colleagues, respecting our own visceral empathy and formulating an intervention plan as soon as possible. At the least, one or two friendly colleagues can approach the physician and share their concerns. They can make time to talk, offer helpful suggestions and resources, and facilitate a referral. They can do this without needing to know with certainty just what the problem might be.

If this intervention is rejected or proves to be unhelpful, the physician must be confronted in a definitive manner. Two or more individuals, respected by the physician and in a position of authority, must intervene in a timely, planned and rehearsed way. They should offer their observations of concern, preferably in documented form, and firmly request an expert clinical assessment—or immediate treatment, if the physician acknowledges a problem. They must not be allowed to manage this alone.

Time away from clinical duties or other work will often be required, both to enable the physician to recover and to ensure patient safety. The physician must be supported every step of the way, and should be reassured of their value as a professional and a person. The desire to return to training or work can in itself motivate a physician to seek the necessary treatment. Finally, the consequences of not complying with the intervention conditions—such as the termination of training or a report to regulatory authorities—must be clearly understood.

Provincial physician health programs are good resources for the planning of interventions and identification of expert assessment and treatment resources.

Outcome

Excellent treatment programs comprising detoxification, education on the mechanisms of dependence, coaching on relapse prevention skills, group support and resources for family members are available for physicians with substance dependence. Inpatient residential treatment is often preferred for physicians but intensive outpatient programs can be effective as well.

With proper treatment and monitoring of recovery, long-term success as measured by abstinence rates and disease remission can exceed 85 per cent (Brewster 2008). Successfully treated physicians not only remain abstinent, but learn about living in a more balanced way. Recovery from substance use disorders means improved physical, psychological, social, familial, occupational and even spiritual health.

It falls to each physician to protect the well-being of their colleagues, to be watchful for signs of drug and alcohol problems, and to be prepared to respond.

Case resolution

The resident's colleague alerts the chief resident and program director of her concerns discreetly. They immediately meet with the resident and request that they proceed to the emergency room for an assessment. The resident complies, and it becomes clear that the resident is intoxicated. The physician health program is notified, and arrangements are made for an urgent assessment. The resident is placed on medical leave. After several months of treatment, the resident is able to return to work, participate in treatment services and health monitoring, and enjoy a full recovery. The physician health program offers to conduct a course for earlier stage intervention as this resident's condition should have been identified and diagnosed by their colleagues sooner.

Key references

Kaufmann M. 2002. Physician substance abuse and addiction: Recognition, intervention and recovery. *Ontario Medical Review*; October 2002; 43-7.

D. Caring for colleagues: Practical issues

Dianne Maier, MD FRCPC

Objectives

This chapter will

- describe the inherent challenges of caring for physician colleagues as patients,
- outline an approach to managing the care of physician patients, and
- discuss physicians' responsibility to care for their colleagues.

> **Case**
>
> A second-year resident is stunned to receive a complaint about the care offered to a physician patient in the emergency department the week before. The patient had presented with chest pain in the context of a recent history of angina and a strong family history of cardiac disease. The physician patient reported that the resident was abrubt, judgemental and dismissive during their encounter. The physician patient complained that history was cursory, the diagnosis brief and the discharge planning suboptimal. The resident remembered the encounter and indicated that, since the patient was a physician, the resident did not feel the need to explain the assessment or treatment recommendations as with other patients.

Introduction

Whether you call it "physicians for physicians," "doctors helping doctors," or "extending professional courtesy," caring for colleagues is an important tradition in medicine. But the thoughtful physician appreciates William Osler's frequently quoted maxim that "The physician who treats himself has a fool for a patient."

Within our current medical culture there is clear endorsement of the following:

- Physicians should seek appropriate medical care, which is not in the corridor or the physician's lounge.
- Physicians should have a family physician and an age-appropriate health assessment as an occupational health imperative: prevention and early intervention are important.
- Physicians should not self-medicate through self-prescribing, the sample cupboard or workplace supplies.

Robert Klitzman has invited physicians to be aware of "post-residency disease" symptoms of which include minimizing and denying symptoms, worrying too little, self-diagnosing and self-prognostication. Physicians worry about the transformation from physician to patient. At times, particularly if they have not experienced or practised being a regular patient, they are confronted by fundamental issues of meaning, identity, work, worsening disease, hope and mortality at such times (Klitzman 2008). Yet, they provide good physician-patient relationships and relationship-centred care for their patients. Physicians should allow themselves to experience that same gift from their own health care providers.

Being a physician-provider

The treating physician and the physician patient can both contribute challenges to good care. The treating physician may feel anxious or intimidated. Perhaps the physician patient in other circumstances was their teacher, or has an impressive reputation for a particular area of expertise. Physician-providers are encouraged to draw upon Richard Frankel's model of communication in health care and consider the following when providing care to a colleague (Maier 2008):

1. Invest in the beginning of the visit. Breathe and remember that an important part of developing rapport is setting the context of the new relationship.
2. Elicit the patient's concerns and listen without interrupting at first. As with other patients, the most important concern may only be brought up after the third concern is presented.
3. Don't assume that physician patients need less explanation than others. Remember that a physician's knowledge of therapeutics in an area of practice not his or her own quickly become dated after medical school.
4. Intellectualizing for your own self-comfort or being drawn into talking shop is not in the best service of your patient.
5. Elicit the perspective of the physician patient. They may have specific ideas or concerns that are not shared by other patients. What does it mean to replace the white coat for the blue gown? (Maier 2008). What does it mean to "immigrate to the nation of the sick?" (Spiro and Mandell 1998). It cannot be assumed physicians will manage the thought or reality of illness better than others. The impact on their ability to keep working may be a particular concern. For example, not all physicians are financially sound or have overhead and/or disability insurance.
6. Get to know the physician patient as a person.
7. Thoroughness, including a complete physical examination, cannot be sacrificed. Physicians are observant and expect physical examinations to be done well. This is beyond technique. It provides comfort and trust in the physician–patient relationship. Technology will never replace it.
8. The demonstration of empathy is as important as in other physician–patient relationships. When we are physicians to colleagues we need to be aware of our own reactions. Is our physician patient's response to illness close to home? Does it influence our care of the physician patient?

9. The end of the visit should involve more than education, involvement in decision-making and enquiring whether your patient got what they needed. As treating physicians we need to be clear and explicit about our practice with regard to prescriptions, consultations and investigations. Discuss who makes the changes and the arrangements. Do not download the physician roles and responsibilities to your physician patient.
10. We all deserve confidentiality and privacy in our health care. However, we may also need to reflect with our physician patient on how privacy issues or maintaining secrets might interfere with the delivery of good health care.
    a. This may be especially relevant when physician patients are suffering from diseases of degeneration (including aging), psychiatric illness or substance use disorders.
    b. We must be aware that illness is not unprofessional conduct and that there is a difference between illness and impairment.
    c. We know that appropriate, early intervention and treatment are as effective for physicians as they are for the general population.
    d. Therefore, if you are unsure about how to assist your physician patient from the perspective balancing the best interest of your patient with your ethical obligations concerning patient safety, consult your provincial physician health program without delay.

In caring for our colleagues we would do well to remember the words of Rabia Elizabeth Roberts: "We learn that our humanity is more powerful than our expertise alone" (Hanlon 2008).

Richard Gunderman would invite us to adopt our part of the highway and to care for one another as colleagues the best way we can. By practising the best kind of philanthropy; the result will benefit the health of all our patients.

Case resolution

The program director reviewed some of the key principles involved in treating colleagues and the importance of maintaining appropriate roles and boundaries in such relationships—professionalism and the value of communication. The resident acknowledged being irritable, fatigued and hungry that evening after being on call again, and having an earlier request to the on call attending in the emergency room for a second opinion refused. The resident and program director discussed a mutually agreeable approach to address the complaint. The resident met with the patient, apologized, and reflected on the frustration, fear, and disappointment the patient had experienced. As a result, the resident gained a deeper level of competence.

Key references

Hanlon V. 2008. Physicians for physicians: when doctors become patients. *Alberta Doctors' Digest.* July/August.

Maier DB. 2008. Physicians for physicians: a call for action. *Alberta Doctors' Digest.* May/June: 18–9.

Spiro HM and HN Mandell. 1998. When doctors get sick. *Annals of Internal Medicine* 128 (2): 52–4.

E. Coping with and respecting the obligations of mandatory reporting

Canadian Medical Protective Association

Objectives

This chapter will

- discuss physicians' ethical and legal obligations with regard to reporting colleagues or physician patients to a regulatory agency,
- outline the consequences of a failure to report, and
- identify sources of support to guide decision-making in this area.

> **Case**
>
> A third-year resident involved in treating a surgeon in Manitoba is aware that the surgeon suffers from alcohol dependence and occasionally experiences tremors and blackouts. The resident suggests that the surgeon not perform any further surgeries until the necessary treatment is obtained. The surgeon continues to practise medicine, but has assured the resident that they do not drink or take drugs before performing surgeries. What are the resident's obligations in the circumstances?

Introduction

Reporting another physician to a medical regulatory authority (college) or public health official can be difficult and stressful, particularly for postgraduate trainees or those who supervise them. Nevertheless, physicians may have ethical and legal obligations to make a report if a colleague's mental or physical health, conduct or behaviour is raising reasonable concerns about his or her ability to practise or is posing a risk to patient safety or public health.

Residents may become aware of these concerns in the course of treating other physicians or through day-to-day contact with colleagues. This section is intended to help residents cope with the stress that arises from uncertainty about their obligations to report impairment in their colleagues.

Reporting a physician who is your patient

In certain circumstances, physicians may have an ethical duty to report the health status of a physician colleague whom they are treating when the condition could reasonably impair that physician's ability to practise or might threaten the safety of patients, staff or others. Various provinces and territories have also enacted legislation that legally requires physicians to report a colleague to their governing college in circumstances when health issues render the physician patient unfit to practise. This may occur when the physician patient refuses to follow recommended and reasonable treatment, such as medications, safety precautions or a leave of absence. A dilemma may arise in these circumstances between the treating physician's duty of confidentiality and the duty to protect the public.

All provinces and territories have public health legislation requiring physicians to report to public health officials patients who have certain communicable diseases, such as AIDS or hepatitis. If a physician is diagnosed with a reportable condition, the treating physician is required to report the case to the individual or office designated in the legislation. Residents who are being treated for serious health issues must also consider whether they are obligated to self-report pursuant to any applicable college policy. A number of colleges include questions on licence applications or renewal forms pertaining to alcohol or drug dependence and any physical or mental conditions that might affect fitness to practise. The Canadian Medical Protective Association (CMPA) can provide members with more information in these circumstances.

Reporting a physician who is not a patient

Residents may also have an ethical and legal duty to report a colleague to their governing college in certain circumstances, such as when health issues render a physician unfit to practise. The triggering criteria vary considerably between jurisdictions. Most statutes and policies require the reporting physician to have reasonable grounds for reporting. Terms such as incompetence, incapacity or unfit are commonly used in this context but are not typically defined in the pertinent statute or policy document.

Reporting concerns about the conduct of a physician

Some jurisdictions have adopted specific reporting requirements for certain conduct issues, such as suspected sexual impropriety by another physician toward a patient. Such an obligation most often arises when the physician has reasonable grounds, based on information obtained in their medical practice, to believe that another physician (whether a patient or colleague) has sexually abused a patient. Some colleges have also adopted policies imposing mandatory reporting obligations in such cases. Physicians should be familiar with the legislation and/or college policies in their province/territory and are encouraged to contact the CMPA in this regard.

All physicians also have an ethical duty to report unprofessional conduct by other physicians, including so-called disruptive behaviour, to an appropriate authority in the institution, often the chief of the department. Physicians may also have a duty to report unprofessional conduct exhibited by a colleague to their governing college. The Canadian Medical Association's *Code of Ethics* states that physicians are ethically bound to report "to the appropriate authority any unprofessional conduct by colleagues."

Deciding to report

In most jurisdictions the duty to report health issues or sexual impropriety applies even when the information became known through a physician–patient relationship, to which a duty of confidentiality would otherwise apply.

When the decision has been made to report, the resident in most cases should first inform the physician that they are obliged to make a report to the college and/or public health officials. The report should then be made as promptly as possible. Concerns regarding a colleague's fitness to practice, incapacity or disruptive behaviour can be particularly stressful for residents. Where appropriate, the resident might offer advice about access to available treatments. The physician who is the subject of the report may be counselled to cease practising in the interim. Generally, avoiding surprises for the physician patient or the colleague and demonstrating support or empathy will assist in easing the tension in these circumstances.

Concerns about exposure to liability and/or college complaints

The failure to report when relevant circumstances exist may result in disciplinary proceedings against either or both physicians. It could also result in a legal action, especially where an individual is allegedly harmed as a result of a physician's incapacity, health status or behaviour.

Although a decision to report may cause considerable angst to a resident, it may be reassuring to know that legislation and the common law generally protect reporting physicians against liability in such circumstances. This legislated protection typically prohibits the commencement of an action against the reporting physician when the report has been made in good faith and without malice.

Documentation

It is important to keep detailed records of relevant information leading up to a report being made, including the outcome of discussions with the physician patient or colleague about whom a report is made, with the college, and with public health officials. A contemporaneous record may be helpful if it is alleged that the report was not made in good faith or on reasonable grounds. Such records should be kept by the resident separately from the patient's chart or the hospital's personnel file and in a manner that protects any personal health information included in the report as well as the personal privacy of the physician who is the subject of the information.

Summary

Some jurisdictions have enacted statutes and/or college policies that create a mandatory duty to report where a physician's health might compromise their ability to practise medicine or put the public's health at risk. All jurisdictions have legislation that requires certain communicable diseases to be reported.

Case resolution:

Manitoba's Medical Act requires the resident to make a report to the College if the resident reasonably believes the surgeon: (a) is unfit to practise, incompetent or unethical; or (b) suffers from a mental or physical disorder or illness that may affect his fitness to practise, and continues to practise despite having been counselled otherwise.

In determining whether to report, the resident must assess whether the surgeon can properly perform surgery even if they do not drink or take drugs before a procedure. If the risks of blackouts, tremors or lapses in judgment remain, a duty to report may arise. In that case, the resident should advise the surgeon that there is an obligation to make a report to the College, and the resident should do so as soon as possible. The resident should keep detailed records of the reasons for reporting and of discussions with the College and the surgeon, including the advice to discontinue practising surgeries.

Physicians in every jurisdiction also have an ethical duty to report unprofessional conduct by colleagues.

Residents should be familiar with the various legal and college reporting requirements and expectations unique to their respective jurisdictions. Since these requirements vary between jurisdictions, it is important that residents consult the specific provision or policy document before making a report. Members of the CMPA may wish to contact the Association for advice if they are uncertain about their obligations.

The decision to report can be difficult, particularly for residents. The stress can be greater in cases where the report concerns the conduct or health of a supervisor. A resident in these circumstances may wish to consider seeking confidential advice from a trusted third party, such as their program director or an official of the provincial residents' association. The appropriate person with whom to discuss concerns will depend on the circumstances. In any event, the information disclosed should generally be anonymous and respectful of the confidential nature of any patient information and the physician's personal privacy. Residents are also encouraged to consult the CMPA for advice regarding these sometimes difficult professional obligations.

Key reference

Canadian Medical Association. 2004. *Code of Ethics* [policy]. Ottawa: The CMA.

F. Canada's physician health programs and resources

W. Todd Watkins, MD BSc CCFP for the CMA Centre for Physician Health and Well-Being

Objectives

This chapter will

- present a list of common physician health resources,
- outline the importance, for physicians, of having a family doctor,
- discuss barriers to seeking help, and
- discuss the risks of not seeking help.

Case

A first-year resident is feeling overwhelmed by the stress associated with moving to a new city, starting residency, and being a new parent. The resident realizes that this current behaviour is unsustainable and that it may lead to burn out. In spite of this, the resident feels unable to seek care from family physicians in this city. The resident is afraid that the family physicians will see them as weak, that word will get out and that their reputation will suffer. The resident fears the stigma associated with asking for help, but even more the resident fears the possibility that they will develop a mental illness that will threaten their ability to complete training and allow the resident to support their new family. The resident feels trapped and doesn't know where to safely turn for help.

Introduction

Although the reader may never need the resources of Canada's network of physician health programs and professionals, it is important for every physicians in the country to know support from the world's leaders in physician support and assistance is only a phone call away.

The scenario described in the case example is common. Physicians who see themselves in this story should know that they are not alone. In fact, most physicians feel overwhelmed at certain points in their career. It is critically important for physicians affected by stress or other health issues to be aware of the confidential resources that are available to them and to make use of them early.

Physician health services: A concerted effort

Over the past two decades, Canadian pioneers in physician health have led a charge to educate physicians about coping with the unique challenges they face in marrying a demanding career with the personal vulnerabilities that allow them to excel at their craft. It was not so long ago that physicians felt unable to broach their own health issues, refusing to accept the realities of the stress and anxiety related to practice.

In the past, physicians typically felt unable to reach out for help when they needed it. Barriers have included fear of stigmatization and of regulatory sanctions, and concerns about confidentiality. Some physicians have attempted to cope on their own, using alcohol or drugs, or suffering from stress, chronic overwork, burnout or more serious mental illnesses. This does not need to be the reality any longer. Canada has become a world leader in the approach to physician health. Although most, if not all, physician support programs were initially created to assist physicians with addictions, there has been a tremendous expansion in the support they provide and the breadth of their services. Each program offers a slightly different array of services, but all provide access to the advice and assistance physicians might need. Contact information for physician health programs across the country is summarized in Chapter 11-B.

Recognizing that the needs of physicians were evolving, these programs came together in 2001 to form the Canadian Physician Health Network (CPHN), a forum that brings together program staff, representatives from the Canadian Federation of Medical Students (CFMS), the Canadian Association of Internes and Residents (CAIR), the Canadian Medical Protective Association (CMPA), the Association of Faculties of Medicine of Canada (AFMC) and the Canadian Medical Association (CMA). Through discussion at this table physician needs are assessed, resources and services are enhanced, and support is given to programs in the early stages of their development.

By 2003, the CMA recognized that more needed to be done to support the health of physicians and created the CMA Centre for Physician Health and Well-being to provide national coordination and raise the profile of this important issue for physicians, their families and other stakeholders, including medical educators, governments and employers. It is important to note, however, that the Centre does not provide personal advice for individual physicians. The Centre spent the first few years building partnerships, creating awareness and defining needs. Through its early work, the health of physicians became one of the CMA's top five priority areas.

The success of the physician health community in building awareness of the importance of physician wellness is based on making the link between physician health on the one hand and quality of care and the sustainability of our health care system on the other. It is this emphasis that makes the Canadian approach truly unique. We know that being healthy ourselves leads to better care for our patients and that losing even a single physician from a community can have a devastating impact on access for patients and the well-being of the physicians who are left to fill the void.

The CMA Centre for Physician Health and Well-being has recently developed a new strategic plan to focus attention on leadership, education and research and continues to complement the work of the individual physician health programs and the CPHN. The Centre is acutely aware that, for students and residents, health and well-being are inextricably linked to debt load, support for career decision-making, reasonable work hours and a safe and supportive training and practice environment, and continues to work with student and resident organizations in advocating for improvements in these areas. The Centre also offers a variety of educational resources, including podcasts, face-to-face courses, national and international conferences and access to an online physician health curriculum based at the University of Ottawa (ephysicianhealth.com).

Readers are encouraged to use www.cma.ca/physicianhealth as their personal portal to access educational resources, new research, literature, emerging policies and strategies. This portal also provides ready access to contact information for all of the physician health programs across the country and other related information.

Critical to the success of the Centre's collective efforts to date has been the involvement of the CFMS and CAIR. Both of these organizations were early leaders working at the national level and with their provincial counterparts to develop policies that protect the health and well-being of medical trainees. In 1998, CAIR developed a position paper on resident well-being that continues to serve as a framework for improvements in the medical training environment. Both organizations have also advocated for significant improvements in the availability of disability insurance and have created well-being days as part of undergraduate and postgraduate training programs. Some of the provincial resident associations also have toll free phone lines to assist trainees. It is important for residents to be aware of the services that their provincial associations offer. These associations have designated wellness officers to interact with the physician health community nationally.

Summary

Despite the tremendous progress in physician health awareness that has been made across the country in recent years, much remains to be accomplished. The resident in the case example has the insight to recognize that he is not coping well, and this a critical step. However, he lacks awareness of the nonjudgmental and confidential resources available to him. As a profession, physicians need to continue to stand by their colleagues, to raise awareness of physician health issues, to lead systemic changes to promote healthier and more sustainable careers, and to ensure that the field of physician health is moving in the right direction.

Case resolution

The resident recalls a series of presentations from their final year of medical school regarding a network of personal resources available to physicians. The resident searches the internet and finds the CMA Centre for Physician Health and Well-being (www.cma.ca/physician-health). There, the resident is comforted to learn that this experience is not at all unusual and that there are lots of resources available.

The resident calls the provincial physician health program and shares their concerns about confidentiality and privacy with the intake staff. The resident finds the explanation of policies in this regard very reassuring. The resident is then referred to appropriate care providers in a nearby community.

With a short course of treatment the resident rapidly builds insight into their own behaviour and learns new coping skills. The resident remains in the program and has a refreshed outlook upon their career. The resident establishes a strong patient–physician relationship with a local family doctor and feels confident in the support.

Key references

Canadian Association of Interns and Residents. Last retrieved on August 10, 2009: www.cair.ca

Canadian Medical Association. *Canadian Physician Health Network*. Last retrieved on August 6, 2009: www.cma.ca/physician-health

Canadian Medical Association. *Centre for Physician Health and Well-being*. Last retrieved on August 6, 2009: www.cma.ca/physicianhealth

Peterkin AD. 1998. *Staying Human During Residency Training*. 2nd Edition. Toronto: U of Toronot Press.

Puddester D. 2004. Canada responds: An explosion in doctors' health awareness, promotion and intervention. *The Medical Journal of Australia*. 181(7): 386–7.

Puddester D. 2001. The Canadian Medical Association's policy on physician health and well-being. *Western Journal of Medicine. January:* 174(1): 5–7.

G. Stress and coping

Jean E. Wallace, PhD; and Jane Lemaire, MD FRCPC

Objectives

This chapter will

- describe key findings from a Canadian study of specialty physicians' stress and wellness, and
- consider how these findings may be relevant to the reader's own study and practice of medicine.

> **Case**
>
> A physician is in the third year of an academic consulting practice, after spending five years training to be a gastroenterologist. The physician greatly enjoyed the patient care during residency training, although considerable stress was associated with long work hours and a lack of control over the work schedule. Now the physician who loves the work is finding both familiar and new stressors.

Introduction

As in any profession, there are ups and downs in the practice of medicine. To explore what young physicians should be prepared to expect from their careers, we summarize the dominant themes that emerged from interviews that we conducted with 42 physicians practising medicine in different specialties in a large health region (Wallace and Lemaire 2008). Their insights reflect a range of life and career stages. In the following discussion we identify those features of medical practice that physicians report are the most satisfying and most stressful aspects of their work.

The ups

We asked physicians to identify the parts of their work that they liked or enjoyed the most or that gave them the greatest satisfaction. The five themes that emerged from their responses were:

1. helping patients, improving their patients' situation and/or making a difference in their patients' lives;
2. interacting with patients (and their families) and getting to know them;
3. working with other doctors, medical staff or on a team;
4. accomplishing work tasks and solving problems; and
5. dealing with challenging or complex cases, diagnoses, and treatments.

Two participants in our study provided the following responses:

"I enjoy seeing patients and talking to patients and their families and sorting out problems for people on a fairly regular day-to-day basis [...] So I guess [...] the part that satisfies me the most is being able to do things for people and hopefully at the end of the day improve their life somehow."

"Sometimes you make a primary diagnosis of cancer, so you get to the bottom of it, you get the answer, you deliver bad news, but you can at least give them the information that they need and try to figure out a solution for them, so problem-solving."

Participants were also asked what aspects of their work they would not be willing to change or give up, even though it might make their work easier. Doctors reported that they enjoy the complexity and acuity of patient cases, the variety that stems from different parts of their job, and spending extra time caring for patients or teaching residents. They would not sacrifice these parts of their work for an easier job.

The downs

In describing their work-related stress, many physicians indicated that it often varied considerably and might fluctuate from day to day as a result of a specific triggering event or incident or depending on the components of their work. Three themes predominated:

1. **Workload (volume/pace of work).** Patient load and demands and a multitude of responsibilities, including and beyond direct patient care.
2. **System access issues.** Patient flow problems, long waiting lists, and difficulties providing timely access to services.
3. **Patient issues.** Difficult interactions with patients, uncertainty or difficulties in diagnosing and/or treating patients, and unexpected events.

Some sample comments are:

"I hate making people wait. I hate seeing a waiting room full of people. I know by the time they see me they're going to be angry, 'cause they've had to wait [...] On the other hand, systemically, I can't not make them wait because I have to book so close together, so it's stressful with that sort of thing going on."

"The wait lists, the wait times, the people who, I mean it's not their fault, who keep coming back because it's six months down the road before I can get them in to see somebody. Total waste of time and energy on everybody's part."

"[...] people who have had nasty experiences with health care in the past, either personally or family members, who are very skeptical of the medical profession and really think that we don't do much for people and that makes them difficult to deal with."

Summary

It is important for physicians to recognize which parts of their work they enjoy and which cause them stress. Through this awareness, they can enhance the ups and hopefully learn to better understand the downs—even when they cannot entirely be controlled. Patient care remains the predominant reward for most physicians, and collegial support has been shown to effectively buffer some of their negative work experiences.

Key references

Linzer M, Gerrity M, Douglas JA, McMurray JE, Williams ES, Konrad TR. 2002. Physician stress: results from the Physician Worklife Study. *Stress and Health*. 18: 37–42.

Wallace JE and JB Lemaire. 2008. *Determinants of Physician Well Being: Stage One Report*. Prepared for the Alberta Heritage Foundation for Medical Research and the Calgary Health Region. June 2008.

Wallace JE and J Lemaire. 2007. On physician well-being—You'll get by with a little help from your friends. *Elsevier Social Science & Medicine*. 64: 2565–77.

Case resolution

The physician takes the time to value the many rich patient encounters they have on a day-to-day basis and begins to understand what types of patient encounters cause stress and why. The physician discusses difficult cases and system access issues with colleagues, as the physician recognizes the value of sharing experiences, advice and information. The physician pledges to a twice-yearly meeting with a mentor to consider workload and career commitments, including and beyond direct patient care. The physician also registers for a continuing medical education conference at least yearly to maintain and update clinical skills.

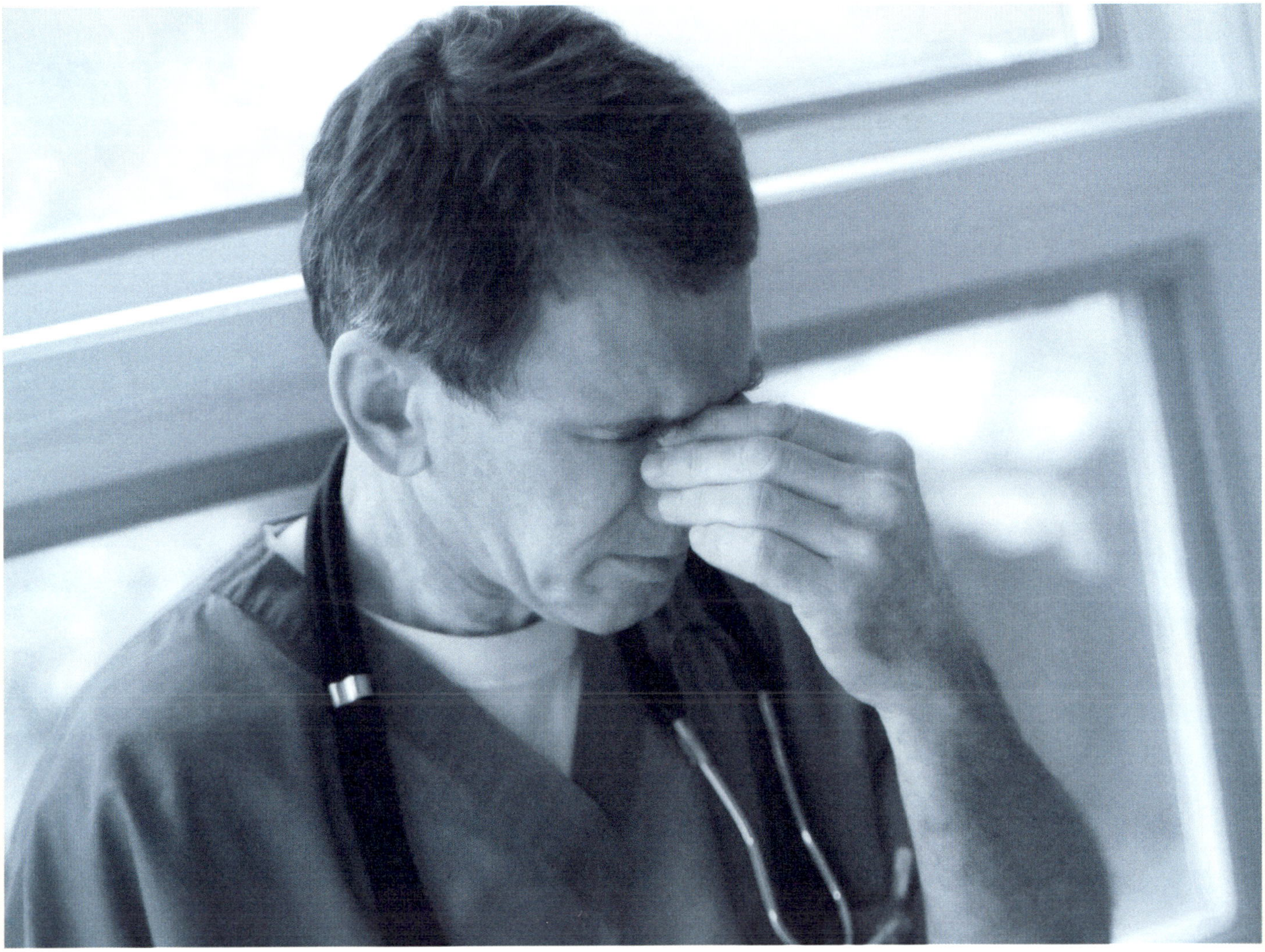

H. Physicians with an illness or a disability

Ashok Muzumdar, MB BS FRCPC

Objectives

This chapter will

- describe some of the unique issues faced by sick or disabled physicians,
- discuss the importance of health promotion and disease prevention in the physician population, and
- identify resources that sick or disabled physicians can use during recovery or their return to training or practice.

> **Case**
>
> A competent and energetic third-year surgical resident has become paraplegic as a result of a motor vehicle accident. After acute care and rehabilitation, the resident regains mobility through the use of a wheelchair. After an absence of eight months, the resident now wishes to return to complete the residency training. This matter is brought before the Department of Surgery. Although there is strong support for the resident on the basis of past performance, there is also some concern. In particular, one senior surgeon expresses doubt about the resident's ability to get to the operating table without the risk of introducing contamination that would compromise patient safety.

Introduction

Because physicians represent a cross-section of society, it should be expected that the illnesses and disabilities that affect the population at large will also occur among physicians. This chapter highlights the impact of physical disability on physicians' professional lives.

The sick physician

Physicians often feel it necessary to project a healthy image of themselves to their patients and colleagues. This attitude can interfere with their ability to acknowledge their own illnesses, and can make it less likely for them to seek independent medical help when they need it.

Physicians reporting to work when they are unwell are likely to compromise their ability to care for their patients properly. Given their professional culture, sick physicians may feel guilty about their illnesses and may be reluctant to take time off work and thereby impose their own workload, including on-call duties, on colleagues. Moreover, a physician may expect the same stoicism on the part of their own colleagues when they are ill. However, physicians who work during an illness may inadvertently put their patients at risk and expose themselves to medical litigation.

Research conducted in Ireland showed that 30 per cent of trainees had not been to a general practitioner within the previous five years, 65 per cent felt unable to take time off when they were ill, and 92 per cent had prescribed themselves medication on at least one occasion. Almost half of participants (49 per cent) felt that they neglected their own health (Uallachain 2007). These findings highlight the need to improve physicians' awareness of their own health needs, beginning early in their careers. The implications of neglecting physician health and well-being can be serious both for practitioners and for patients.

Residents and practising physicians often do not have their own primary care physician. Because of their knowledge of medicine, as well as for the sake of convenience while working long hours, some doctors are prone to self-diagnosing and self-prescribing, notwithstanding the fact that their own illness may not be in their area of medical expertise. Self-diagnosis and self-treatment deny physicians the benefit of an independent, unbiased assessment and care. Various international studies have demonstrated that a high percentage (in the vicinity of 90 per cent in most studies) of trainee and practising physicians self-diagnose and self-medicate from time to time.

The most commonly self-prescribed drugs are analgesics, antibiotics, tranquilizers and hypnotics. Some physicians become habitual self-prescribers. These practises are often acquired early in their training and professional lives. Their program directors need to be cognizant of the possibilities of such risky behaviour, which can in some cases lead to drug dependency and addiction.

Lisa Graves' 2008 article in Medical Teacher observes: "The wounded healer remains easily hidden in a profession that implicitly, and at times actively, encourages a denial of illness. In training, however, the wounded healer can be identified and treated before entering clinical practice. It would seem, then, that medical school and residency is an optimal time to identify and treat the wounded healer." Physicians have a strong sense of responsibility and commitment to their patients, colleagues and community. To fulfill their role in society, it is equally important for them to practise a healthy lifestyle and to seek prompt medical attention when they are sick.

The disabled physician

Although some entrants to medical school have disabilities, it more commonly happens that a physical or mental disability is acquired during the learning years or in subsequent years of medical practice. The impact of the disability will depend on the type of condition, its severity, and its interplay with the environment in which the physician has to function.

Early in training physicians need to be aware that at some point during their lifetime they will encounter unforeseen illness, injury and/or disability. Therefore, it is essential that residents and practitioners alike obtain appropriate expert advice from an insurance professional to provide adequate financial protection for themselves and their families. Physicians report that, after acquiring a disability, new insurance coverage may be impossible to obtain, and may come with unaffordable premiums. Provincial/territorial medical associations offer physician health programs for their members. The Canadian Medical Association's Centre for Physician Health & Well-being is an excellent resource for all physicians.

Disabilities influence to varying degrees a resident or practising physician's ability to continue in their field. A mild disability may have minimal or no adverse functional effect on a physician. A severe disability, such as a major brain injury, may make it impossible for that trainee or physician to return to their training or practice. Notwithstanding these exceptions, most physicians with disabilities should be able to resume their training or return to practice either in the same form or in a modified setting. A disabled resident or physician may find that their program directors and colleagues are willing to offer assistance when and where required and that they demonstrate an understanding of the challenges associated with a disability. However, the trainee or physician may encounter situations in which co-workers are less than sympathetic toward their specific circumstances.

The Canadian Human Rights Act stipulates that employers must provide sufficient accommodation to any worker with a disability. Under the Act, employers are expected to exhaust all reasonable avenues of accommodation, including workplace modification, for an individual with a disability while also taking into account health and safety issues in the workplace. To balance the obligations of a program director/administrator, it is also essential for a resident/physician with a disability to demonstrate that they are able to function safely and to practise competently.

Physicians who wish to return to training or practice after acquiring a disability and can do so competently and safely, working with or without the use of functional aids and essentially on par with their fellow physicians, should be able to do so. They should be given every possible assistance on the part of program directors, colleagues and administrators to facilitate their return to training or practice. Should disabled physicians have any questions or concerns, they should contact the Canadian Medical Protective Association (CMPA) and their respective medical licensing authority for guidance.

The Canadian Association of Physicians with Disabilities (CAPD) is the first organization in the world dedicated to bringing together medical students, residents and practising physicians with any type of physical or mental disability to provide a common forum to lend support to one another, exchange information and advocate on behalf of all persons with disabilities to promote and enhance the interests of the disabled population.

Case resolution

The program director asks the resident to meet to discuss the resident's needs should the resident be allowed to resume training. The resident had already researched the area of work modification. At the meeting the resident requests to be permitted to use a separate "clean" wheelchair for sole use in the operating room (OR) area with a similar protocol applied to the wheelchair as that applied to OR trolleys for transporting patients. To avoid any contamination of the resident's gloved hands and surgical gown, the draped chair would be wheeled from the scrub room to the operating table by an OR assistant. The resident demonstrated the ability to stand and balance quite well with the bilateral long leg braces that had already been prescribed during rehabilitation. These modifications were found to be acceptable, and the resident was able to rejoin training on a trial basis under supervision.

Key references

Graves L. 2008. Teaching the wounded healer. *Medical Teacher*. 30 (2): 217–9.

Uallachain GN. 2007. Attitudes towards self-health care: a survey of GP trainees. *Irish Medical Journal*. 100 (6): 489–91.

Introduction: Financial health

Jordan Cohen, MD FRCPC

Financial worries are one the key sources of stress for resident physicians. These worries may be related to existing debt from undergraduate studies and medical school, the limited salary received during residency, or the effects of poor spending habits. Given the already overloaded schedule of a resident focused on developing clinical proficiency while trying to keep up with many other professional and personal activities, little time may be left to attend to financial matters. Many residents are either too exhausted to consider managing their finances or procrastinate until the end of their training, hoping that life will work itself out. In part, this may be a way of avoiding the stress of dealing with financial concerns. However, it may also be fair to say that many programs and medical schools set their residents up for this stress by not organizing seminars on financial management, not properly advertising or making the resources that are available for financial planning more accessible, and not conveying the importance of setting up a proper financial plan during the training years.

Myths about finances

In considering—or not considering—their financial well-being, residents often make assumptions such as the following:

- I'm going to be independently wealthy when I complete my training, and so I don't need to consider finances now.
- I don't have enough money to pay off my debt or make investments during residency.
- I don't have the time to consider finances during my training.
- I can't afford to eat out, fix my car or go on vacation because of my debt. I'll enjoy these luxuries once I've completed residency.

Residents typically carry an incredible financial load in comparison with non-physicians of the same age. They have been shown to have four times the average debt load, as well as significantly less in savings, than age-matched controls in the general population (Teichman et al 2005). To some extent the debt load of resident physicians may reflect a lack of basic knowledge about financial management. However, it also seems that residents as a group are not effective at budgeting or paying off bad debt such as credit card expenses. Proper financial planning should be considered in much the same way as preventive medicine—that is, as a way to reduce the morbidity of personal debt.

Work habits and specialty choice have been shown to be affected by residents' financial situations. Those with heavy debt often moonlight to supplement their income; however, this extra workload can exacerbate physical and mental stress. Ironically, despite their higher debt and lower savings, many residents do not take advantage of tax-free investing for their futures, such as through registered retirement savings plans (RRSP). Their high levels of debt may be correlated with a lack of budgeting by residents. Studies have concluded that residents do require more teaching around financial planning.

This section will demonstrate with detailed case examples how good financial planning can help to alleviate money worries and secure a better future after residency training. The relevance of financial health to physician health and well-being is discussed, basic terms and concepts in financial management are outlined, and particular attention is given to budgeting and debt management. By giving adequate attention to personal financial management, residents can help to prepare the ground for a secure future.

Checklist for financial planning

- Attend a workshop or seminar on financial planning.
- Read a self-help book on basic personal finances and financial planning.
- Consult a financial planner.
- Before completing your training, attain the services of:
  (1) an accountant,
  (2) a billing clerk,
  (3) a financial planner, and
  (4) possibly a lawyer (for contract negotiations, if applicable to your health region).
- Ask mentors about the strategies they have used to ensure their own financial welfare.
- Budget but don't limit essentials (e.g., proper nutrition) and still treat yourself (e.g. vacations, hobbies).

Key references

Greene AK and M Puder. 2002. A resident's guide to personal finance. *Current Surgery.* 59 (4): 423–5.

Teichman JMH, Cecconi PP, Bernheim BD, Novarro NK, Monga M, DaRosa D, Resnick M and Study Group. 2005. How do residents manage personal finances? *American Journal of Surgery.* 189 (2): 134–9.

A. Financial planning

Magalie Dubé, MD FRCPC

Objectives

This chapter will

- describe the key components and benefits of comprehensive financial planning,
- outline key components of debt management, and
- reflect on the link between financial and personal health.

> **Case**
>
> A fourth-year resident would like to lease a new car but doesn't know if they can afford it. The resident has made a budget, but has trouble sticking to it. The resident feels that they do not have a good grasp of where their money goes. The resident would like to have a better understanding of the basics of financial planning so that they can take better control of this situation.

Comprehensive financial planning

An evaluation of their current and potential financial resources can help individuals develop a plan that will help them to achieve their personal and professional goals and objectives. A certified financial planner (CFP) is a professional who is qualified to assess their clients' financial situation, review their goals and objectives, and recommend an action plan to work toward short- and mid-term goals and long-term aspirations. Ideally, a CFP will also identify when the advice and assistance of other experts, such as accountants, lawyers or insurance brokers are also needed, and will help to coordinate consultations with these advisors.

Comprehensive financial planning can be broken down into six basic steps:

1. Gather information on your current situation.
2. Establish goals and objectives.
3. Analyze your current financial situation.
4. Formulate recommendations.
5. Implement a financial plan.
6. Periodically review and evaluate your progress.

Current situation

You will share with the financial consultant certain personal information (e.g., name, address, date of birth, marital status, number of dependants). You will be asked for other relevant information, such as your banking institution and the contact information of your accountant and lawyer. The financial consultant will make a detailed examination of your present and future finances to prepare the pertinent documents and financial statements that form the basis of your financial plan.

- **Personal financial information.** This will include salary, all sources of income, rent, mortgage, education, car and all other living costs for yourself and your dependants.
- **Statement of net worth.** This is a compilation of your current assets and liabilities; the difference between them represents your equity or net worth.
- **Cash flow statement.** This highlights your cash in flows (sources of income) and outflows (expenses). This analysis of your resources and discretionary spending may help you to find ways to improve your financial position.
- **Statement of insurance requirements.** This analysis allows you to assess whether your life and disability insurance coverage is meeting your goals in securing a source of income replacement for your loved ones in the event of your death, or for you and your dependants in the event that through accident or illness you become unable to earn an income.

Goals and objectives

With the help of your financial planner, you will formulate financial goals and objectives in relation to a measurable time frame.

Analysis

The objective is to find a balance between current finances and future goals. This will mean analyzing existing restrictions on your cash flow and the limitations of your financial position. With the help of a financial consultant you may realize that your current spending habits are working against your long-term goals. The ultimate goal is to find ways to improve cash flow and make appropriate decisions about all the things that are important to you.

Recommendations

After this process of financial analysis, you and your financial consultant will agree on short- and long-term goals. Then, concrete steps and recommendations will be established for you to follow and to monitor, with the support of your financial consultant.

Implementation and follow-up

The steps and activities included in your financial plan should be described and prioritized to help you to understand and follow them. Financial planning is a dynamic process influenced by the professional and personal events that unfold in your life. To reach your long-term goals and have a secure financial future, meet at least once a year with your financial planner.

Case resolution

The resident meets with a CFP recommended by a colleague. Before their first meeting, the CFP provides a sample worksheets to prepare the resident for the questions that will be asked. They establish the resident's statement of net worth as at December 31.

Assets ($)	
Cash	0
Medical library	1,500
Computer	2,500
Used car	5,000
Total	**9,000**
Liabilities ($)	
Credit card debt	500
Line of credit	50,500
Total	**51,000**
Net worth	**$(-42,000)**

Because of the significant debt they accrue during their training, it is the norm, not the exception, for medical residents to have a negative net worth. The purpose of the resident's net worth statement is to take a snapshot of their current financial position that will provide a starting-point for subsequent planning.

The financial consultant then helped the resident to produce an accurate cash flow statement for the previous month.

Cash inflow ($)	
Net salary (after deductions)	**3,150**
Cash outflow ($)	
Rent and utilities	850
Loan repayment	500
Food and entertainment (restaurants)	500
Auto, parking	300
Tuition fees, medical books	100
Clothing	200
Miscellaneous	300
Total expenses	**(-2,750)**
Net cash inflow (outflow)	**$400**

After reviewing life and disability insurance coverage, the financial consultant suggested that the resident meet with an insurance specialist to ensure adequate coverage.

With the help of the CFP, the resident formulated three financial goals and objectives:

- To be free of all training-related debt within five years after residency.
- To purchase a desirable home within the first five years after residency.
- To sell the resident's old car (which is barely working) and use the money to decrease the monthly payment on a new car lease.

In reviewing the cash flow statement, the resident realizes that by spending less on clothing and restaurant meals they would be able to reach these objectives sooner. The resident obtains written financial recommendations and plans to start implementing them in the near future. The financial consultant and the resident have a follow-up meeting in three months to evaluate progress and to address any questions that arise.

Summary

Because of the need to simultaneously manage debt, create cash flow and prepare for the future, professional financial planning is crucial for physicians, particularly in their early years of practice. Contacting and meeting a CFP before the end of the residency will help you to start off on the right foot.

Key references

Canadian Medical Association. *CMA Practice Management Curriculum Modules for Medical Residents. Module 2: Financial Planning.* Last retrieved on August 10, 2009: www.cma.ca/index.cfm/ci_id/39363/la_id/1.htm#module_2.

B. Debt management

Magalie Dubé, MD FRCPC

Objectives

This chapter will

- discuss the burden of debt typically incurred by medical residents, and
- describe basic approaches to managing debt.

> **Case**
>
> A resident who will be completing training in six months and their spouse, who is also in the last year of residency, don't have any children yet and live in a condominium owned by the resident's in-laws. The resident has accumulated $60,000 in debt (on a personal line of credit) during training and has $20,000 in student loans. The resident's spouse has $25,000 in student loans and a line of credit of $40,000. They both have good credit ratings.

Introduction

In 2007, the average debt of Canadian medical residents at the end of training was reported as $158,728 (Kondro 2007). Indeed, given rising tuition costs, debt during medical training has become a necessary evil for most residents. However, not all debt is the same, and proper debt management can lower overall interest payments and help to speed up repayment.

The most frequent types of debt incurred by medical residents are:

- Canada and provincial student loans,
- unsecured liability such as lines of credit and loans from a bank or other financial institution,
- car loans, and
- consumer or credit card debt.

Most residents have acquired some type of government indebtedness during their school years, such as loans negotiated with federal and/or provincial student loan authorities. This debt tends to be relatively favourable in terms of after-tax rates and repayment options. However, interest on Canada Student Loans starts to accrue upon completion of medical school, before the recipient is earning a significant income. Several Canadian provinces have therefore pioneered programs to defer interest on the provincial portion of medical resident loans.

The interest rates on federal and provincial student loans may be as high as two or three percentage points above the prime lending rate. However, the interest paid on these loans has been claimable as a federal tax credit since 1998. Most provinces provide such tax credits as well. A certified financial planner (CFP) can be of great service in assessing the value of these tax credits relative to the benefit of loan consolidation.

It has been quite easy for medical students and residents to obtain lines of credit from a bank or financial institution. Even though most people pursuing a career in medicine will need some form of unsecured credit during their training, this should be monitored closely, and proper short- and long-term financial planning should be in place. Ideally, an application for a line of credit or an increase to a line of credit should be discussed beforehand with a financial planner.

The interest rate on unsecured loans offered to medical students and residents can be as low as the prime lending rate if the applicant has a good credit rating. Interest rates on secured liabilities such as a car loans are usually higher, ranging from two to three percentage points above the prime lending rate. The most expensive form of debt is consumer indebtedness accrued through credit card purchases. Here, interest rates can vary from 16 to 24 per cent of the balance, depending on the client's credit rating. Paying down a credit card balance by using a personal line of credit can save 11 to 19 per cent of the interest on purchases per year.

Pros and cons of student loan consolidation

All physicians can claim a federal tax credit (15 per cent in 2008) on payments of the interest portion of outstanding loans obtained through the Canada Student Loans Program, provincial or territorial loans programs, or both. Interest paid for any other indebtedness, such as bank loans or lines of credit, are not eligible for this credit.

Debt repayment and RRSP contributions

Retirement objectives should be part of the discussion of long-term goals with a financial planner. Beginning the retirement saving process early in one's career has significant advantages, and contributing to a registered retirement savings plan (RRSP) is a great place to start. However, residents who are carrying a significant debt load and are faced with a limited cash flow may wonder about the relative merits of paying down their debt versus contributing to a RRSP. Although a CFP can help to calculate the financial benefits of each alternative, the final decision may be a matter of personal preference and of risk tolerance. Learning how different financial management practises can best fit a residents personal level of comfort and current financial situation can lead to a significant decrease in stress and improve well-being.

Negotiating with financial institutions

Residents can save precious time and avoid unnecessary frustration by working with a financer who is familiar with physicians' particular needs and concerns, understands the generalities of their training, is knowledgeable about their current and future income potential, and is able to structure products for their individual needs. As a professional group, physicians benefit from terms that are more advantageous than those normally negotiated by individuals. A financial consultant can provide their physician clients with some useful advice in preparation for a meeting with a financial institution's account manager.

Credit rating

The term "credit rating" refers to the assessment of an individual's ability to repay debt in a timely manner. A credit rating is based mainly on an individual's history of debt repayment, his or her current financial position (assets and liabilities) and likely future income. Because banks often place more emphasis on current credit rating than on future income potential, it is crucial to maintain an excellent credit rating. Credit reporting agencies such as Equifax (www.equifax.ca), TransUnion (www.transunion.ca) and Northern Credit Bureaus (www.credit-bureau.ca) collect, store, analyze and sell such information. Because credit ratings are based on a seven-year cycle, any late interest payments or failures to pay bills will have a negative impact on an individual's credit rating for some time. It is worthwhile to check one's credit rating at least yearly to correct any errors that might appear on one's record. A financial consultant can provide advice on maintaining a good credit rating.

Case resolution

The resident, and spouse, seek financial advice to help choose a debt management strategy and evaluate their options with respect to RRSPs.

Good debt management involves evaluating all liabilities with respect to type of debt, amount, interest and conditions of repayment. Many young physicians wisely approach their financial institutions to consolidate their loans into a line of credit or term loan. With good credit ratings, they can negotiate a line of credit at interest rates as low as the prime lending rate. Debt consolidation not only saves money but can also free up cash flow to reduce indebtedness and accelerate repayment.

However, caution should be used when considering consolidating Canada or provincial/territory student loans. Interest paid on these debts is entitled to a federal and provincial tax credit on your tax return. With the help of a financial consultant, the resident compares the after-tax cost of each scenario.

The bank offers the resident and spouse the prime rate of four per cent on a line of credit to consolidate their indebtedness—including their student loans, on which they have been paying prime plus three per cent. The bank's offer seems to be attractive, but after a closer look, the actual after-tax savings would be approximately 1.25 per cent. In consolidating all debts to the bank, the residents will forfeit both federal and provincial tax credits. If the student loans stay outside of the loan consolidation, the residents will realize an after-tax interest rate of approximately 5.25 per cent per annum (i.e. 7 per cent less approximately 25 per cent combined in federal and provincial interest tax credits).

The financial planner gave three alternatives to the residents on their debt management process.

Focus on savings: If they both purchase $13,000 of RRSPs per year for five years, they could have at the end of the period $130,000 (plus interest) in RRSPs but would still have $145,000 of indebtedness. Net worth of ($15,000).

Focus on reducing debt: After four years of practice the $145,000 of debt would be paid, but no RRSP assets would be owned. Net worth of $0.

Combine strategies: By combining these strategies, seven years after beginning practice they could eliminate the debt ($145,000) but have RRSP assets of $55,000. Net worth of $55,000.

A good financial planner can give you options and help you decide on an action plan that respects your attitude and preferences. Understanding the pluses and minuses of consolidating loans, repaying debt, purchasing retirement savings plans is important for all residents who wish to plan for their financial future. Trainees should be proactive with their money by negotiating with financial institutions and improve credit rating. Through appropriate financial planning all residents can secure financial health.

Key reference

Canadian Medical Association. 2008. *Tax Tips for the Medical Student, Resident and Fellow.* Ottawa: The CMA.

Kondro W. 2007. Debt woes [newsbrief]. *Canadian Medical Association Journal.* 176: 919.

A. Further reading and additional references

1-D. Physician health: A business case

Canadian Institute for Health Information. 2007. *Supply, Distribution and Migration of Canadian Physicians, 2007.* Last retrieved June 24, 2009: secure.cihi.ca/cihiweb/dispPage.jsp?cw_page=AR_14_E.

Canadian Medical Association. 2003. *Stressors Unique to Medicine.* Last retrieved June 24, 2009: www.cma.ca/index.cfm/ci_id/25573/la_id/1.htm.

Cohen J. 2004. *"Happy Doc" Study Surveys Residents Nationwide. In Creating a Healthy Culture in Medicine: a Report From the 2004 International Conference on Physician Health.* Ottawa. CMA Centre for Physician Health and Well-Being.

College of Family Physicians of Canada, Canadian Medical Association, Royal College of Physicians and Surgeons of Canada. 2008. *Medical Student and Resident Data Backgrounder of the 2007 National Physician Survey (NPS).* Last retrieved June 24, 2009: www.nationalphysiciansurvey.ca/nps/news/PDF-e/NPS%20-%20Student%20&%20Resident%20Backgrounder.pdf

College of Family Physicians of Canada, Canadian Medical Association, Royal College of Physicians and Surgeons of Canada. 2007. *National Physician Survey.*

Epstein RM. 2003. Virtual physicians, health systems, and the healing relationship. *Journal of General Internal Medicine.* 18 (5): 404–6.

Frank JR, Brien S, (Editors) on behalf of The Safety Competencies Steering Committee. 2008. *The Safety Competencies: Enhancing Patient Safety Across the Health Professions.* Otawa, ON: Canadian Patient Safety Institute.

Gautam M and WT Watkins. 2008. *Physician Morale and Medical Workplace—A Canadian Perspective. Canadian Medical Association* paper for International Medical Workforce Collaborative Conference.

Jovic E, Lemaire J, Wallace JE. 2006. The generation and gender shifts in medicine: an exploratory survey of internal medicine physicians. *BMC Health Services Research.* Last retrieved June 24, 2009: www.biomedcentral.com/1472-6963/6/55.

Klie S. 2008. Sick and tired in the workplace. *Canadian HR Reporter.* June 2.

Lemaire J and JE Wallace. 2008. Physician wellness. *Parkhurst Exchange.*

Lemaire J and JE Wallace. 2007. On physician well-being—You'll get by with a little help from your friends. *Elsevier Social Science & Medicine.* 64: 2565–77.

Logan C, Director Disability Services, Homewood Employee Health: personal conversation

Padmos A. 2008. *Message from the CEO: Patient Safety.* Last retrieved June 24, 2009: rcpsc.medical.org/about/CEO/Message_from_CEO_oct08_e.pdf.

Quality Worklife—Quality Healthcare Collaborative. 2007. *Within Our Grasp—A Healthy Workplace Action Strategy for Success and Sustainability in Canada's Healthcare System.* Ottawa: Canadian Council on Health Services Accreditation.

Rich P. 2008. Complex care for complex patients in a complex time. *MDPulse.*

Wilkerson B. 2008. *The Health of Physicians is Key to a Healthy Economy and a Healthy Nation* [presentation]. Global Business and Economic Roundtable for Mental health

1-E. Societal Expectations

Brown JB, Sangster LM, Østbye T, Barnsley JM, Mathews M, Ogilvie G. 2002. Walk-in clinics: patient expectations and family physician availability. *Family Practice.* 19 (2): 202–6.

Wilkerson B. 2009. The health of physicians is key to a healthy economy and a healthy nation. *Global Business and Economic Roundtable on Addiction and Mental Health.* Last retrieved June 24, 2009: www.mentalhealthroundtable.ca

2-B. Reflective practice

Mamede S and HG Schmidt. 2004. The structure of reflective practice in medicine. *Medical Education.* 38 (12): 1302–8.

Novack DH, Suchman AL, Clark W, Epstein RM, Najberg E, Kaplan C. 1997. Calibrating the physician. Physician personal awareness and effective patient care. *Working Group on Promoting Physician Personal Awareness, American Academy on Physician and Patient. Journal of the American Medical Association.* 278 (6): 502–9.

2-C. Emotional intelligence

Gardner H. 2000. *Intelligence Reframed: Multiple Intelligences for the 21st Century.* New York: Basic Books.

Goleman D. 2000. *Working with Emotional Intelligence.* New York: Bantam Books.

A. Further reading and additional references

Mayer JD, author, Brackett MA, Salovey P, eds. 2004. *Emotional Intelligence: Key Readings on the Mayer and Salovey Model.* New York: Dude Publishing.

2-D. Leadership and leadership skills

Roberts LW. 2009. Leadership in academic psychiatry: the vision, the "givens," and the nature of leaders. *Academic Psychiatry.* 33 (2): 85–8.

Waldhausen J. 2001. John H. Gibbon, Jr., lecture: Leadership in medicine. *Bulletin of the American College of Surgeons.* 86 (3):15–9.

3-Introduction: Balancing personal and professional life

Canadian Medical Association. 1998. *Physician Health and Well-being* [policy]. Ottawa: The CMA.

Frank E. 2004. Physician health and patient care. *Journal of the American Medical Association.* 291: 637.

Frank E, Breyan J, Elon L. 2000. Physician disclosure of healthy personal behaviors improves credibility and ability to motivate. *Archives of Family Medicine.* 9: 287–90.

Frank E, Hedgecock J, Elon LK. 2004. Personal health promotion at US medical schools: A quantitative study and qualitative description of deans' and students' perceptions. *BMC Medical Education.* 4: 29.

Paice E, Rutter H, Wetherell M, Winder B, McManus IC. 2002. Stressful incidents, stress and coping strategies in the pre-registration house officer year. *Medical Education.* 36: 56–65.

Puddester D. 2001. The Canadian Medical Association's policy on physician health and well-being. *Western Journal of Medicine.* 174: 5–7.

Shanafelt TD, Sloan JA, Habermann TM. 2003. The well-being of physicians. *The American Journal of Medicine.* 114: 513–9.

Taub S, Morin K, Goldrich MS, Ray P, Benjamin R, for the Council on Ethical and Judicial Affairs of the American Medical Association. 2006. Physician health and wellness. *Occupational Medicine.* 56: 77–82.

3-A. Maintaining relationships during training and beyond

Armstrong A, Alvero R, Dunlow S, Nace M, Baker V, Stewart E. 2009. Balancing the professional and personal. *Journal of Fertility and Sterility.* 91 (1): 18–21.

3-B. Promoting healthy partnerships in medical families

Gabbard GO and RW Menninger. 1989. The psychology of postponement in the medical marriage. *Journal of the American Medical Association.* 261 (16): 2378–81.

Gottman JM and N Silver. 1999. *The Seven Principles for Making Marriage Work.* New York: Three Rivers Press.

Hill M and N Love. 2008. Medical relationships: practice guidelines. *Physician and Family Support Program presentation 2008/2009.* Presented in Edmonton: Sturgeon Medical Staff Retreat, April.

Maier DB. 2005. Hope you are reading this on the beach … . *Alberta Doctors' Digest.* July/August.

Maier DB. 2005. Mama doc, papa doc. *Alberta Doctors' Digest.* January/February.

Maier DB. 2003. Physician mistakes spouse as an employee. *Alberta Doctors' Digest.* May/June.

Myers MF. 1994. *Doctors' Marriages: A Look at the Problems and Their Solutions.* 2nd ed. New York: Springer-Verlag.

Rubin D. 2006. Balancing family and career: addressing the challenges facing dual-career couples. *Gastrointestinal Endoscopy* 63 (6): 831–3.

Schrager S, Kolan A, Dottl SL. 2007. Is that your pager or mine: a survey of women academic family physicians in dual physician families. *Wisconsin Medical Journal.* 106 (5): 251–5.

Sobecks NW, Justice AC, Hinze S, Taylor Chirayath H, Lasek RJ, Chren MM, et al. 1999. When doctors marry doctors: a survey exploring the professional and family lives of young physicians. *Annals of Internal Medicine.* 130 (4, pt 1): 312–9.

Straehley C and P Longo. 2006. Family issues affecting women in medicine, particularly women surgeons. *American Journal of Surgery.* 192: 695–8.

Warde C, Allen W, Gelberg L. 1996. Physician role conflict and resulting career changes: gender and generational differences. *Journal of General Internal Medicine.* 11: 729–35.

4-A. Mindfulness and stress management

Benson H. 1975. *The Relaxation Response.* New York: Avon Books.

A. Further reading and additional references

Hanh TN. 1975. *The Miracle of Mindfulness: A Manual on Meditation*. Boston: Beacon Press.

Tolle E. 1997. *The Power of Now: A Guide to Spiritual Enlightenment*. Vancouver: Namaste Publishing Inc.

4-B. Journal writing

DasGupta S. 2006. How to catch the story but not fall down: Reading our way to more culturally appropriate care. *Virtual Mentor*. 8 (5): 315–8.

Charon R. 2006. The self-telling body. *Narrative Inquiry*. 16 (1): 191–200.

Frank AW. 1995. *The Wounded Storyteller: Body, Illness, and Ethics*. Chicago: University of Chicago Press.

4-C. Exercise and physical fitness

Abramson S, Stein J, Schaufele M, Frates E, Rogan S. 2000. Personal exercise habits and counseling practices of primary care physicians: A national survey. *Clinical Journal of Sport Medicine*. 10: 40–8.

Haskell WL, Lee IM, Pate RP, Powell KE, Blair SN, Franklin BA, et al. 2007. Physical activity and public health: Updated recommendation for adults from the *American College of Sports Medicine and the American Heart Association. Circulation*. 116: 1081–93.

Warburton DER, Nicol CW, Bredin SSD. 2006. Prescribing exercise as preventive therapy. *Canadian Medical Association Journal*. 174: 961–74.

4-D. Spirituality

Chodron P. 1997. *When Things Fall Apart: Heart Advice for Difficult Times*. Boston: Shambhala Publications.

Koenig HG, McCullough ME, Larson DB. 2001. *Handbook of Religion and Health*. New York: Oxford University Press.
Remen RN. 1997. *Kitchen Table Wisdom: Stories That Heal*. New York: Riverhead Books.

Richmond L. 1999. *Work as a Spiritual Practice: A Practical Buddhist Approach to Inner Growth and Satisfaction on the Job*. New York: Broadway Books.

Steindl-Rast D. 1984. *Gratefulness, the Heart of Prayer: An Approach to Life in Fullness*. New York: Paulist Press.

Wilber K. 1997. *The Eye of Spirit: An Integral Vision for a World Gone Slightly Mad*. Boston: Shambhala Publications.

4-E. Finding a family physician

Black D. 2000. POM + EBM = OPD? *Journal of Medical Ethics*. 26: 229–30.

Charles C, Whelan T, Gafni A. 1999. What do we mean by partner in making decisions about treatment? *BMJ*. 319: 780–2.

Gilsdorf JR. 2006. *Inside/Outside: A Physician's Journey With Breast Cancer*. Ann Arbor: University of Michigan Press.
Groopman J. 2007. *How Doctors Think*. New York: Houghton Mifflin Company.

Klitzman R. 2007. *When Doctors Become Patients*. New York: Oxford University Press.

Tyssen R. 2007. Health problems and the use of health services among physicians: a review article with particular emphasis on Norwegian studies. *Industrial Health*. 45: 599–610.

4-F. Nutrition

Faugier J, Lancaster J, Pickles D, Dobson K. 2001. Barriers to healthy eating in the nursing profession: Part 1. *Nurse Standard*. 15 (36): 33–6.

Faugier J, Lancaster J, Pickles D, Dobson K. 2001. Barriers to healthy eating in the nursing profession: Part 2. *Nurse Standard*. 15 (37): 33–5.

Firth-Cozens J, Greenhalgh J. 1997. Doctors' perceptions of the links between stress and lowered clinical care. Social Science & Medicine. 44 (7): 1017–22.

Health Canada. *Dietary Reference Intakes*. Updated Jan 10, 2004. Last retrieved June 25, 2009: www.hc-sc.gc.ca/fn-an/nutrition/reference/index-eng.php.

Health Canada. *Eating Well with Canada's Food Guide*. Updated Dec 20, 2007. Last retrieved June 25, 2009: www.hc-sc.gc.ca/fn-an/food-guidealiment/index-eng.php.

Lemaire J and JE Wallace. 2006. *Seeking Balance Study: The Final Report*. Calgary: Department of Medicine, University of Calgary.

Lemaire J, Wallace JE, Dinsmore K, Lewin A, Ghali W, Roberts D. 2009. Physician nutrition and cognition during work hours: Effect of a nutrition based intervention. *Unpublished Manuscript*.

A. Further reading and additional references

Parshuram CS, Dhanani S, Kirsh JA, Cox PN. 2004. Fellowship training, workload, fatigue and physical stress: A prospective observational study. *Canadian Medical Association Journal.* 170 (6): 965–70.

Shirom A, Nirel N, Vinokur AD. 2006. Overload, autonomy, and burnout as predictors of physicians' quality of care. *Journal of Occupational Health Psychology.* 11 (4): 328–42.

5-A. Determinants of workplace health

Cottingham AH, Suchman AL, Litzelman DK, Frankel RM, Mossbarger DL, Williamson PR, et al. 2008. Enhancing the informal curriculum of a medical school: a case study in organizational culture change. *Journal of General Internal Medicine.* 23 (6): 715–22.

Mareiniss DP. 2004. Decreasing GME training stress to foster residents' professionalism. *Academic Medicine.* 79 (9): 825–31.

Peterkin AD. 2008. *Staying Human During Residency Training: How to Survive and Thrive After Medical School.* 4th ed. University of Toronto Press Thomas NK. 2004. Resident burnout. *Journal of the American Medical Association.* 292 (23): 2880–9.

Shapiro SL, Shapiro DE, Swartz GER. 2000. Stress management in medical education: a review of the literature. *Academic Medicine.* 75 (7): 748–59.

5-D. Professionalism: Reasonable expectations

Baldwin DC Jr, Daugherty SR, Rowley BD. 1998. Unethical and unprofessional conduct observed by residents during their first year of training. *Academic Medicine.* 73: 1195–200.

Cruess SR and RL Cruess. 2000. Professionalism: a contract between medicine and society. *Canadian Medical Association Journal.* 162: 668–9.

Gruen RL, Pearson SD, Brennan TA. 2004. Physician-citizens — public roles and professional obligations. *Journal of the American Medical Association.* 291: 94–8.

Hilton SR and HB Slotnick. 2005. Proto-professionalism: how professionalisation occurs across the continuum of medical education. *Medical Education.* 39: 58–65.

Levinson W and N Lurie. 2004. When most doctors are women: What lies ahead? *Annals of Internal Medicine.* 141: 471–4.

Lopez L and JT Katz. 2009. Perspective: creating an ethical workplace: reverberations of resident work hours reform. *Academic Medicine.* 84: 315–9.

Swick HM. 2000. Toward a normative definition of medical professionalism. *Academic Medicine.* 75: 612–6.

Working Party of the Royal College of Physicians. 2005. Doctors in society. Medical professionalism in a changing world. *Clinical Medicine.* 5 (6 suppl 1): S5–40.

Wynia MK, Latham SR, Kao AC, Berg JW, Emanuel LL. 1999. Medical professionalism in society. *New England Journal of Medicine.* 341: 1612–6.

5-F. Intimidation and harassment in training

Cohen JS and S Patten. 2005. Well-being in residency training: a survey examining resident physician satisfaction both within and outside of residency training and mental health in Alberta. *BMC Medical Education.* 5: 21.

Quine L. 2003. Workplace bullying, psychological distress, and job satisfaction in junior doctors. *Cambridge Quarterly of Healthcare Ethics.* 12: 91–101.

Stebbing J, Mandalia S, Portsmouth S, Leonard P, Crane J, Bower M, Earl H, Quine L. 2004. A questionnaire survey of stress and bullying in doctors undertaking research. *Postgraduate Medical Journa*l. 80: 93–6.

Tibbo P, de Gara CJ, Blake TM, Steinberg C, Stonehocker B. 2002. Perceptions of intimidation in the psychiatric educational environment in Edmonton, Alberta. *Canadian Journal of Psychiatry.* 47: 562–7.

Zweibel EB and R Goldstein. 2001. Conflict resolution at the University of Ottawa Faculty of Medicine: the pelican and the sign of the triangle. *Academic Medicine.* 76 (4): 337–44.

6-Introduction: Collegiality

Janus K, Amelung VE, Baker LC, Gaitanides M, Schwartz FW, Rundall TG. 2008. Job satisfaction and motivation among physicians in academic medical centers: insights from a cross-national study. *Journal of Health Politics, Policy and Law.* 33 (6): 1133–67.

Madsen TE and DR Martin. 2006. Resident perception of a newsletter's impact on residency morale and collegiality. *Medical Education Online* [serial online]. 11: 22.

Stark R, Korenstein D, Karani R. 2008. Impact of a 360-degree professionalism assessment on faculty comfort and skills in feedback delivery. *Journal of General Internal Medicine.* 23 (7): 969–72.

A. Further reading and additional references

6-B. Conflict management

Fisher R. 1977. *Resolving Interpersonal Conflict.* Rev. 2000. School of International Service: The American University. Last retrieved August 10, 2009: www.aupeace.org/files/Fisher_ResolvingInterpersonalConflict.pdf

McKay M, Davis M, Fanning P. 1995. *Messages: The Communication Skills Book.* 2nd ed. Oakland: New Harbinger Publications.

Thomas KW and RH Kilmann. 2009. *Thomas-Kilmann Conflict Mode Instrument.* Mountain View,: CPP Inc.

6-E. Interdisciplinary relationships

Bulgar RJ and RE Bulgar. 1992. Obstacles to collegiality in the academic health centre. *Bulletin of the New York Academy of Medicine.* 68 (2): 303–7.

Canadian Medical Association. 2008. *Achieving Patient Centered Collaborative Care* [policy]. Ottawa: CMA.

Goldstein M. 1992. Maintenance of collegiality. *Bulletin of the New York Academy of Medicine.* 68 (2): 308–13.

Huffman M. 1993. Family physician and the healthcare team. *Canadian Family Physician.* 39: 2165–70.

Jensen PM, Trollope-Kumar K, Waters H, Everson J. 2008. Building physician resilience. Canadian Family Physician. 54 (5): 722–9.

Salvage J and R Smith. 2000. Doctors and nurses doing it differently. *BMJ.* April 15;320 (7241) 1019-20.

The American College of Physicians Manual: ACP Ethics Manual, Professionalism Charter. Last retrieved August 13, 2009: www.acponline.org/ethics/ethics man.htm

Zelek B and S Phillips. 2003. Gender and power: Nurses and doctors in Canada. *International Journal of Equity in Health.* 2:1

7-Introduction: Physician health and the doctor–patient relationship

Hall KH. 2001. Sexualization of the doctor–patient relationship: Is it ever ethically permissible? *Family Practice.* 18: 5115.

Hughes J. 1994. The doctor–patient relationship: a review. In *Organization and Information at the Bed-Side.* Chicago: University of Chicago.

Myers M. 2005. Finding a doctor can be the toughest challenge — even for a doctor. In *Creating a Healthy Culture in Medicine: A report from the 2004 International Conference on Physician Health.* Ottawa: CMA Centre for Physician Health and Well-being.

7-B. Coping when values collide

Cantor J and K Baum. 2004. The limits of conscientious objection—May pharmacists refuse to fill prescriptions for emergency contraception? *New England Journal of Medicine.* 351 (19): 2008–12.

Savulescu J. 2006. Conscientious objection in medicine. *BMJ.* 332: 294–7.

Sulmasy DP. 2008. What is conscience and why is respect for it so important? *Theoretical Medicine and Bioethics.* 29 (3): 135–49.

Wicclair MR. 2008. Is conscientious objection incompatible with a physician's professional obligations? *Theoretical Medicine and Bioethics.* 29 (3): 171–85.

7-C. Coping with challenging patient behaviour

Shusterich KM. 1990. Helping physicians manage challenging patient encounters–Part 1. *Physician Executive.* 16 (6): 26–9.

Shusterich KM. 1991. Helping physicians manage challenging patient encounters. Part 2—Improving physician–patient relationships from an administrative point of view. *Physician Executive.* 17 (1): 20–2.

7-D. Boundary issues

College of Physicians and Surgeons of Ontario. 2008. *Maintaining Appropriate Boundaries and Preventing Sexual Abuse* [policy #4-08]. Last retrieved June 25, 2009: www.cpso.on.ca/policies/policies/default.x?id=1604&terms=maintaining+appropriate+boundaries+and+preventing.

College of Physicians and Surgeons of Ontario. 2004. Maintaining boundaries with patients. *Members' Dialogue.* September/October.

Schoener GR. 1998. Boundaries in professional relationships. *Advocate Web.* Last retrieved June 25, 2009: www.advocateweb.org/home.php?page_id=48.

8-A. Major transitions

Baker NJ. 1992. Maternity leave for practicing family physicians. *Journal of Family Practice.* 35 (1).

A. Further reading and additional references

Deeson JD. 2006. Have you planned for physician succession & retirement? *Physician's Weekly*. 23 (14).

Faulkner LR. 2007. Personal reflections on a career of transitions. *Journal of the American Academy of Psychiatry and the Law Online*. 35: 253–9.

Gautam M and R MacDonald. 2001. Helping physicians cope with their own chronic illnesses. *Western Journal of Medicine*. 175 (5): 336–8.

McCall MW Jr and JA Clair. 1992. In transit from physician to manager–part I. *Physician Executive*. 18 (2): 3–9.

9-A. Physical health

Canadian Physician Health Network. Last retrieved June 25, 2009: www.cma.ca/index.cfm/ci_id/25567/la_id/1.htm.

Dubey V, Mathew R, Katyal S, Iglar K. *The Evidence-Based Preventive Care Checklist Form*. The the College of Family Physicians of Canada. Last retrieved August 14, 2009: www.cfpc.ca/English/cfpc/communications/health%20policy/Preventive%20Care%20Checklist%20Forms/Intro/default.asp?s=1

Gilsdorf JR. 2006. *Inside/Outside: A Physician's Journey with Breast Cancer*. Ann Arbor: University of Michigan Press.

Groopman J. 2007. *How Doctors Think*. New York: Houghton Mifflin Company.

Institute for Clinical Systems Improvement. [website]. Last retrieved on August 14, 2009: www.icsi.org

Klitzman R. 2007. *When Doctors Become Patients*. New York: Oxford University Press.

Tyssen R. 2007. Health problems and the use of health services among physicians: a review article with particular emphasis on Norwegian studies. *Industrial Health*. 45: 599-610.

9-C. Substance use, abuse and dependence

Baldisseri MR. 2007. Impaired healthcare professional. *Critical Care Medicine*. 35 [Suppl]: S106-16.

Brewster JM, Kaufmann IM, Hutchison S, MacWilliam C. 2008. Characteristics and outcomes of doctors in a substance dependence monitoring programme in Canada: A prospective descriptive study. *BMJ*: 337. a2098

Hughes PH, Brandenburg N, Baldwin DC, Storr CL, Williams KM, Anthony JC, Sheehan DV. 1992. Prevalence of substance use among US physicians. *JAMA*: 267(17). 2333-9

9-D. Caring for colleagues: Practical issues

Frankel RM, Stein T, Krupat E. 2003. *The Four Habits Approach to Effective Clinical Communication*. Oakland: Kaiser Permanente.

Goldman LS, Dickstein LJ, Myers M. 2000. *The Handbook of Physician Health: The Essential Guide to Understanding the Health Care Needs of Physicians*. Chicago: American Medical Association.

Gunderman R. 2008. Resilience in personal and professional life [presentation]. *Alberta Psychiatric Association* meeting, Apr 4, Banff, Alta.

Hurst JW. 2003. What do good doctors try to do? *Archives of Internal Medicine*. 163: 2681–6.

Klitzman R. 2008. *When Doctors Become Patients*. New York: Oxford University Press.

Myers MF and GO Gabbard. 2008. *The Physician as Patient: A Clinical Handbook for Mental Health Professionals*. Arlington: American Psychiatric Publishing.

Roberts E. 2007. Showing up: notes on action in the world. *Desert Call*. Winter: 4–7. In Hanlon V. 2008. Physicians for physicians: when doctors become patients. *Alberta Doctors' Digest*. July/August.

9-G. Stress and coping

Arnetz BB. 2001. Psychosocial challenges facing physicians of today. *Social Science and Medicine*. 52: 203–13.

Dunstone DC and HR Reames. 2001. Physician satisfaction revisited. *Social Science and Medicine*. 52: 825–3

Dyrbye LN, Thomas MR, Shanafelt TD. 2006. Systematic review of depression, anxiety, and other indicators of psychological distress among U.S. and Canadian medical schools. *Academic Medicine*. 81 (4): 354–73.

Firth-Cozens J. 2001. Interventions to improve physicians' well being and patient care. *Social Science and Medicine*. 52: 215–22.

Keeton K, Fenner DE, Johnson RB, Hayward RA. 2007. Predictors of physician career satisfaction, work-life balance, and burnout. *Obstetrics and Gynecology*. 109: 949–55.

A. Further reading and additional references

Shanafelt TD, Sloan JA, Haberman TM. 2003. The well-being of physicians. *American Medical Journal.* 114: 513–9.

9-H. Physicians with and illness or disability

Canadian Association of Physicians with Disabilities. www.capd.ca.

Canadian Medical Association Centre for Physician Health & Well Being. www.cma.ca/physicianhealth.

Canadian Medical Protective Association. www.cmpa-acpm.ca.

B. Provincial and national resources

National physician health program

CMA Centre for Physician Health and Well-being

877 CMA-4-YOU (877 262-4968)
cma.ca

Provincial physician health programs

Physician Health Program of British Columbia

Toll free: 1-800-663-6729
604-742-0747
info@physicianhealth.com
www.physicianhealth.com

Alberta Physician and Family Support Program

Toll free: 1-877-767-4637
Program/administration office phone: 403-228-2880
Program/administration office toll free: 1-877-262-7377
pfsp@albertadoctors.org
www.albertadoctors.org, Under Benefits and Services

Saskatchewan Physician Support Program

Toll free: 1-800-667-3781 (in province only)
306-244-2196
SPSP committee members as listed in the "members only" section of the website
brenda@sma.sk.ca
www.sma.sk.ca

Manitoba Physician at Risk Program

204-237-8320

Physician Health Program, Ontario Medical Association

Toll free: 1-800-851-6606 (in province)
Toll free: 1-800-268-7215 x2972 (rest of Canada)
michael_kaufmann@oma.org , cynthia_macwilliam@oma.org
www.phpoma.org

Quebec Physicians' Health Program

Toll free: 1-800-387-4166
514-397-0888
info@pamq.org
www.qphp.org

Nova Scotia Professional Support Program

902-468-8215
robert.fredrickson@doctorsns.com
jan.goodwin@doctorsns.com
professionalsupport@doctorsns.com

New Brunswick Physician Health Program

Toll free: 1-888-453-7272 (24-hour voice messaging)
Messages returned daytime hours Monday to Friday
New Brunswick Medical Society: 506-458-8860
lricharddespres@nbms.nb.ca
www.nbms.nb.ca

Prince Edward Island Physician Support Program

Toll free: 1-877-626-3955 (within 902 area code)
902-626-3955
airwin@mspei.org
www.mspei.org

Newfoundland Professionals' Assistance Program

Toll free: 1-800-563-9133
709-754-3007
rmlahey@nl.rogers.com
www.nlpap.ca

Other resources

University of Ottawa Faculty Wellness Program

613-562-5800 x8507
wellness@uottawa.ca
www.medicine.uottawa.ca/wellness

Canadian Association of Internes and Residents

613-234-6448
cair@cair.ca
www.cair.ca

Canadian Federation of Medical Students

613-565-7740
office@cfms.org
www.cfms.org

Fédération des médecins résidents du Québec

Toll free: 1-800 465-0215
514-282-0256
fmrq@fmrq.qc.ca
www.fmrq.qc.ca

C. Online and e-resources

The Royal College of Physicians and Surgeons of Canada CanMEDS resources

The CanMEDS 2005 Physician Competency Framework
rcpsc.medical.org/canmeds/CanMEDS2005/index.php

The CanMEDS Assessment Tools Handbook
rcpsc.medical.org/canmeds/resources/handbook_e.php

CanMEDS Best Practices
rcpsc.medical.org/canmeds/bestpractices/index.php

Bibliography of CanMEDS Competencies
rcpsc.medical.org/canmeds/bestpractices/bibliography_e.php

The Royal College of Physicians and Surgeorns of Canada CPD Program Guide
rcpsc.medical.org/opd/cpd/prog-guide_e.pdf

CMA resources

Canadian Physician Health Network
www.cma.ca/index.cfm/ci_id/25567/la_id/1.htm

Doctors' Health Matters: Finding the Balance.
Report from the 2008 International Conference on Physician Health
www.cma.ca/multimedia/CMA/Content_Images/Inside_cma/Physician_Health_and_Wellbeing/physician_health_conference/PHWB-2008conf-report_e.pdf

Physician Health and Well-being
CMA Policy
policybase.cma.ca/dbtw-wpd/PolicyPDF/PD98-04.pdf

Creating a Healthy Culture in Medicine
Report of the 2004 AMA/CMA International Conference on Physician Health
www.cma.ca/multimedia/CMA/Content_Images/Inside_cma/Physician_Health_and_Wellbeing/English/healthy-culture.pdf

A Physician's Guide to Coping with Death and Dying
www.cma.ca/index.cfm/ci_id/43636/la_id/1.htm

The Non-financial Aspects of Physician Retirement:
Environmental Scan & Literature Review
www.cma.ca/multimedia/staticcontent/CMA/Content_Images/Inside_cma/Physician-Health/English/pdf/Retirement-lit-summary.pdf

CMA Guide to Physician Health and Well-Being
www.cma.ca/multimedia/staticContent/HTML/N0/l2/PhysicianHealth/resources/guide-PHWB.pdf

CMA Code of Ethics
policybase.cma.ca/PolicyPDF/PD04-06.pdf

Rural and Remote Practice Issues
CMA Policy
policybase.cma.ca/dbtw-wpd/PolicyPDF/PD00-08.pdf

Additional online resources

ePhysicianhealth.com

eWorkplacehealth.com

Foundation for Medical Excellence
www.tfme.org

Physician Health and Well-being
Physicians' Guide to the Internet
physiciansguide.com/dochlth.html

The Centre for Professional Well-being
www.cpwb.org

Centre for Professional Health
Vanderbilt Medical Centre
www.mc.vanderbilt.edu/root/vumc.php?site=cph

Healthy and active living

Healthy living
Heart and Stroke Foundation Canada
www.heartandstroke.com/site/c.ikIQLcMWJtE/b.3483949/k.967D/Healthy_Living.htm

Eating well with Canada's food guide
www.hc-sc.gc.ca/fn-an/food-guide-aliment/index-eng.php

Physical Activity Guides
www.hc-sc.gc.ca/hl-vs/physactiv/index-eng.php

The Vitality Approach: A Guide for Leaders
Health Canada
www.hc-sc.gc.ca/fn-an/nutrition/weights-poids/vitalit/vitality_approach-approche_vitalite-eng.php

C. Online and e-resources

Healthy workplaces

Lowe GS. *Are Healthy Workplaces More Productive?* 2003.
www.cprn.org/doc.cfm?doc=299&l=en

Framework for Development of a Healthy Workplace.
National Quality Institute.
www.nqi.ca/nqistore/Product_details.aspx?ID=70

Faculty wellness

Faculty Wellness Program.
University of Ottawa
www.medicine.uottawa.ca/wellness/eng/terms.html

Medical students

Canadian Federation of Medical Students
www.cfms.org

Canadian Medical Association's Med Student Centre
www.cma.ca/index.cfm/ci_id/121/la_id/1.htm

American Medical Student's Association's Medical Student Well-Being
www.amsa.org/well

Residents and interns

Canadian Association of Interns and Residents
www.cair.ca

CAIR position papers on Resident Well-being
www.cair.ca/document_library/docs/Wellbeingpaper.pdf

Fédération des médecins résidents du Québec (FMRQ)
www.fmrq.qc.ca/formation-medicale/index.cfm

Women in medicine

Federation of Medical Women of Canada
www.fmwc.ca

Rural physicians

Society of Rural Physicians
www.srpc.ca/mainframe.html

Rural Canadians, Health Canada
www.hc-sc.gc.ca/hl-vs/jfy-spv/rural-rurale-eng.php

Sexual orientation

Gay and Lesbian Medical Association
www.glma.org

Association of Gay and Lesbian Psychiatrists
www.aglp.org

Aboriginal people

Institute for Aboriginal Health
www.iah.ubc.ca

Visions
www.visions.ab.ca

First Nations, Inuit & Aboriginal Health, Health Canada
www.hc-sc.gc.ca/fniah-spnia/index-eng.php

Public Health Agency of Canada
www.phac-aspc.gc.ca/chn-rcs/aboriginal-autochtones-eng.php

Racial groups

Racism in the medical profession: the experience of UK graduates (BMA, June 2003)
www.bma.org.uk/employmentandcontracts/equality_diversity/ethnicity/racism.jsp

Physicians with disabilities

Canadian Association of Physicians with Disabilities
www.capd.ca

Physicians' families

Kid's Help Phone
www.kidshelpphone.ca

D. Templates for reaching out

Derek Puddester, MD MEd FRCPC

Concerned about a trainee?

1. Be sure your concern is reasonable, objective as possible, and valid.

2. Learn about the supports trainees can utilize locally, provincially, and nationally. If you're not sure, speak to your local health/ wellness resources or your provincial physician health program. A listing can be found at www.cma.ca/physicianhealth. You can learn more about health and wellness issues for physicians at www.ephysicianhealth.com as well.

3. Plan a private meeting with the trainee. Emphasize that the meeting is meant to be supportive, a mutual sharing of concern, and involving mutual brainstorming about next steps.

4. State your concern simply and clearly. Invite their response and perspective.

5. If there is agreement, invite suggestions for intervention. Share the information from the relevant portions of this guide as well as contact information for clinical supports.

6. Acknowledge that you are not in a role to act as their physician and ignore all urges to diagnose and treat. Leave this to the individual's clinician.

7. Offer them time off to attend to their health, your ongoing support, and your willingness to help them move forward.

8. If your concerns involve patient care and safety consider your duty to the public as well as the trainee. If you are not sure, speak to the CMPA for advice.

9. If the learner is not meeting academic expectations or if your concerns involve patient care/safety, consider a mandatory independant medical evaluation (IME). Your PHP can help organize these for you. Be prepared to cover all costs involved and also be reasonable in your expectations of the report. In general, you will only receive relevant diagnosis/recommendations in an effort to respect the privacy of the learner.

10. If you feel the trainee is at imminent risk of self harm or harm to others state your concern clearly and request they present to the emergency room. If this is not successful, consider alerting the police.

11. Be prepared to support a well-planned medical leave.

12. Welcome residents back to training in the context of the approval of their clinicians, appropriate documentation of health, a thoughtful return-to-work plan, and consideration of ongoing monitoring of health.

D. Templates for reaching out

Derek Puddester, MD MEd FRCPC

If you are a program director and are concerned about the morale and health of your program:

1. Reflect carefully on your leadership, that of your committee, and the overall culture of your Department.

2. Procure an external consultant to collect qualitative and quantitative data about the health and wellness of your program.

3. Invite them to present their findings to the entire Department in a transparent fashion.

4. Consider the tools required to shift culture in your group. These may involve healthy policies that are actually implemented (e.g. intimidation and harassment, conflict management, evaluation and promotion), educational sessions focused on skill development (e.g. communication, self-care, emotional intelligence, generational differences).

If you are a resident and are concerned about your own health:

1. Visit your family physician and fully share your concerns.

2. Consider their recommendations carefully, including investigations/treatments and follow-up.

3. Avoid the temptation to self-diagnose or treat.

4. Do not ask fellow trainees or supervisors to diagnose/treat.

5. Call your local health and wellness programs - they can often help you find a family physician or other clinical/non-clinical supports.

6. Call your Provincial Physician Health Program.

7. Consider options such as taking a health leave or training part-time as part of your recovery.

8. Seek and accept support from friends, family and colleagues. Avoid the urge to isolate.

9. Practice healthy behaviours as much as possible - monitor the basics (sleep, nutrition, hydration, recreation, intimacy) and practice principles of sustainability.

E. Useful strategies for coping with long work hours

Jason R. Frank, MD MA(Ed) FRCPC

Maintain Rhythms

1. Circadian rhythms (e.g., good sleep hygiene)
2. Social rhythms (e.g., family time)
3. Psychological rhythms (e.g., weekly schedule)
4. Physical rhythms (e.g., regular exercise routine)

Counteract Fatigue

1. Adequate regular sleep
2. Judicious caffeine
3. Avoiding alcohol and other drugs
4. Breaks, naps, and variety
5. Exercise
6. Bright light

Manage Time Effectively

1. Knowing yourself.
2. Prioritizing and setting goals.
3. Following a plan.
4. Getting organized.
5. Leveraging resources.

Engaging Others

1. Educate loved ones about medical work
2. Ensure decision-makers understand the nature of medicine

Revitalize

1. Take holidays and plan the next one
2. Destress
3. Focus on activities outside medicine
4. Take time to reflect
5. Reassess personal values and priorities

F. Quick reference index

Highlighted here are some of the most common terms used to discuss issues of physician health and the pages where these terms are discussed throughout the text.

